Viva Voce in ORTHODONTICS

Other CBS titles by the same author

Short Notes for Dental PG Entrance Examinations, Vol I
❖ Chronology ❖ Orthodontics ❖ Endodontics ❖ Local Anaesthesia
❖ Dental Histology ❖ Embryology ❖ Oral Pathology and Medicine ❖ Radiography

Short Notes for Dental PG Entrance Examinations, Vol II
❖ Anatomy ❖ Physiology ❖ Dental Anatomy ❖ Biochemistry ❖ Microbiology
❖ Dental Materials ❖ Fluorides and Community Dentistry ❖ Pharmacology

Short Notes for Dental PG Entrance Examinations, Vol III
❖ All remaining topics

***MCQs in Dental Sciences:* National Boards of USA and Canada**

Viva Voce in ORTHODONTICS

SANDEEP GOYAL MDS (Orthodontics)
Reader, Department of Orthodontics and Dentofacial Orthopedics, MM College of Dental Sciences and Research, Mullana, Ambala, Haryana

Formerly
Resident, KGMC, Lucknow
Registrar, PGIMS, Rohtak
Reader, DAV (C) Dental College, Yamuna Nagar

Edited by

Sonia Goyal MDS (Oral and Maxillofacial Surgery)
Senior Lecturer, Department of Oral and Maxillofacial Surgery, M. M. College of Dental Sciences and Research, Mullana, Ambala, Haryana

CBS

CBS PUBLISHERS & DISTRIBUTORS
NEW DELHI • BANGALORE

Viva Voce in ORTHODONTICS

First Edition : 2004
Reprint : 2005

ISBN : 81-239-1095-9

Publishing Director : Vinod K. Jain

Published by :
Satish Kumar Jain for CBS Publishers & Distributors,
4596/1-A, 11 Darya Ganj, New Delhi - 110 002 (India)
E-mail : cbspubs@del3.vsnl.net.in
Website : http://www.cbspd.com

Branch Office :
Seema House, 2975, 17th Cross, K.R. Road,
Bansankari 2nd Stage, Bangalore - 560070
Fax : 080-6771680 • E-mail : cbsbng@vsnl.net

Typeset at CBS P&D Typesetting unit and printed at
Asia Printograph, Shahdara, Delhi - 110032 (India)

dedicated to

my

parents

Acknowledgement

At the very outset, I bow my head to almighty God for his blessings and giving me the opportunity to work.

I cannot forget the sacrifices of my parents who worked very hard to make me educated. Without their constant encouragement, I was not able to complete this work.

My wife, Dr Sonia, has always stood by me during the tough time, and this is due to her immense help and constant support that I am able to bring this work to its present form.

I am highly indebted to my teachers, viz. Dr D N Kapoor, Ex-Professor & Head, Department of Orthodontics, Faculty of Dental Sciences, KGMC, Lucknow; Dr V P Sharma, Professor & Head, Department of Orthodontics, Faculty of Dental Sciences, KGMC, Lucknow; and Dr Pardeep Tandon, Professor, Department of Orthodontics, Faculty of Dental Sciences, KGMC, Lucknow, for all their support, advice and words of encouragement during my post-graduation, that I could achieve this rare feat now.

I acknowledge Dr Sanjay Tiwari, professor and head of Department of Endodontics, GDC, Rohtak, for his constant support and encouragement.

My big brother, Amit, needs special words of thanks at this juncture, for it is his effort which has enabled me to work incessantly and I could be able to complete the work.

I wish to thank Mr. S K Jain, managing director, and Mr Y N Arjuna, publishing director, CBS Publishers and Distributors, and their team of experts, whose invaluable efforts presented the work in the best possible form.

Lastly, I wish to thank all my family members for their unending support.

Dr Sandeep Goyal

Suggested Readings

1. Graber's
2. Graber and Swain
3. Profitt's
4. White and Gardeiner
5. C.P Adams
6. Chakona's
7. Gianelley's
8. Skinner's
9. Thurow's
10. Moyer's
11. Andersean's
12. Petrovic's
13. Graber's and Neumann's
14. W J Clark's

Preface

There has always been a lacuna of a good book for preparing for *viva voce* for the dental students since a long time. A lot many standard books are available in the market on the subject of orthodontics, but all those books are not able to answer the small queries of the students. However, these books, if read sincerely, are the best guides for understanding the subject, but at undergraduate level the student is not that much experienced so as to grab the points written in them.

This book has been compiled with this idea in mind so as to solve the queries of the undergraduate student to the best possible extent. Its format of questions and the short answers lends itself to the dissemination of the information as was always desired by the students. The format also permits a lack of formality not available in the standard textbooks. The goal of this work is to provide what the readers will enjoy and find useful and stimulating. The important points have been compiled in tabular form and also sometimes repeated in the text for continuous revision for the students.

This book is not a substitute for the standard textbooks available in the field of orthodontics as written by the experienced orthodontists. Thereby, it is suggested that the student should pursue the additional readings in the areas of his interest. While short answers provide the passage of succinct information, they do not allow for much discussion. It has been tried to explain the questions sufficiently to meet the needs of the dental students.

It has been requested in my other books, viz ***Short Notes for Dental PG Entrance Examinations :*** Vols 1–3, and ***MCQs in Dental Sciences,*** that the feed-back from the readers is the best remedy to improve upon the work in future. So, I again request you all to give your invaluable suggestions and contribution towards the improvement of the book for the benefit of future dentist and orthodontists.

I thank my wife Dr Sonia Goyal for editing and making her significant contribution in the preparation of the manuscript of this book.

Dr Sandeep Goyal

Contents

1

General Orthodontics

◎ Define orthodontics?

According to British Society of Orthodontics, 1922 "Orthodontics includes the study of the growth and development of the jaws and face particularly, and the body generally as influencing the position of the teeth; the study of action and reaction of internal and external influences on the development and the prevention and correction of arrested and perverted development."

◎ What are the branches of orthodontics?

It has been divided in 4 branches as follows:

1. Preventive orthodontics
2. Interceptive orthodontics
3. Corrective orthodontics
4. Surgical orthodontics

◎ What do you mean by preventive orthodontics?

These are the actions taken to preserve the integrity of what appears to be the normal occlusion at a specific time.

◎ Define interceptive orthodontics?

It is the phase of the science and the art of orthodontics to recognize and eliminate the potential irregularities and malpositions in the developing dentofacial complex. These are the procedures done at an early stage of a malocclusion to eliminate or reduce the severity of the same.

◎ Define corrective orthodontics?

Orthodontic actions taken to correct a fully developed and established malocclusion.

◎ What is surgical orthodontics?

These are the procedures undertaken as an adjunct to the orthodontic treatment. It also involves the correction of dentofacial deformities of the severe nature which cannot be treated by orthodontics alone. However, these should be done only after the completion of growth phase to avoid the future relapse tendency.

◎ What are the aims of orthodontic treatment?

These are functional efficiency, structural balance and esthetic harmony. It is also aka **Jackson's triad**.

◎ When should be the orthodontic treatment started?

There is not any specific time to start the orthodontic treatment. It depends on the severity of the condition and its influence on the dentofacial complex. There are certain conditions which require treatment as early as possible. For example, anterior or posterior cross bites, as any delay in their treatment can lead to the increase in the severity of the condition or the skeletal growth. However, the severe skeletal class III malocclusion is best treated after all the skeletal growth is completed by surgical management.

◎ Who is the father of orthodontics?

Kingsley is the father of orthodontics; while Angle is the father of modern orthodontics. Orthodontics is the first and the oldest speciality of dentistry.

◎ Who is the father of cephalometry?

Broadbent and Hoffrath in 1931 devised the cephalostat although independently, and has been considered the fathers of cephalometry.

Reader's Notes

2

Growth and Development

BASIC CONCEPTS

◎ **What do you mean by Growth?**

It is an increase in size.

◎ **What do you mean by Development?**

It is the progress towards maturity, i.e. growth + differentiation + translocation.

◎ **What is the amount of the Height Increase?**

Height increases by 5000 folds in the prenatal period as opposed to only 3-fold increase during the entire postnatal period.

◎ **What are the factors affecting the Physical Growth?**

Various factors are heredity, nutrition, illness, race, socioeconomic factors, family size, birth order (first child has less birth weight and stature but more IQ), secular trends, food habits, exercise and climate.

◎ **What is the meaning of the term Differentiation?**

It is a change from generalized cell to a specialized kind, i.e. a change in quality.

◎ **What is the meaning of Maturation in context of the Growth?**

It expresses the qualitative changes which occur with age.

◎ **What is the Translocation of the Bone?**

It is **passive** growth of bone. It is a ***change in the position*** of whole bone. It depends on capsular matrix and is aka *displacement* of the bone.

◎ **What are the components of the Primary Growth?**

It is actual **translation** (passive growth) and remodelling of bones.

◎ **What do you mean by Secondary Growth?**

It is the **transformation** (periosteal) + sutural growth.

◎ **What do you mean by Transformation?**

It is **active** growth. It is the apposition and resorption in a bone. It is a local change and occurs under the influence of periosteal matrix, and is aka the apposition and resorption in a bone.

◎ **What do you mean by the Intrinsic Genetic Factors and the Epigenetic Factors?**

Intrinsic genetic factors mean those factors, which are inherent in the skull tissues themselves. The epigenetic factors mean that these factors are genetically determined, but manifest their influence in an indirect way by intermediary action on the associated structures (eye, brain, etc.). Modification of these soft tissues has a modifying effect on the primary craniofacial complex.

◎ **What are the different Mechanisms of Bone Growth?**

a. **Bone deposition and resorption** = known as **bone remodelling.**
b. **Cortical drift** = combination of bone deposition and resorption resulting in a *growth movement towards the depository surface*.
c. **Displacement** = is the *movement of whole bone as a unit*. It is due to pull or push of different soft and bone tissues as they all continue to enlarge.
d. **Primary or active displacement** = i.e. if bone gets displaced due to its own growth. For example, growth at maxillary tuberosity pushes maxilla anteriorly.

e. **Secondary or passive displacement** = i.e. if the bone gets displaced due to growth and enlargement of an **adjacent bone**.

f. **Sutural growth.**

g. **Enlow's expanding V–principle** = many bones / parts of the bone have V–shape pattern of the growth, which occurs towards wider ends of the V due to selective apposition and resorption.

h. **Enlow's counterpart principle** = states that the growth of any given facial or cranial part relates specifically to other structural and geometric counterparts in face and cranium.

i. **Neurotrophism** = is a non-impulse transmitting neural function which involves axoplasmic transport and provides for long term interaction b/w neurons and innervated tissues, which homeostatically regulates the morphological, compositional and functional integrity of these tissues.

◎ What are the different periods of prenatal growth and development?

It has been studied in 3 phases viz.

1. Period of ovum 0–2 wks of i.u. age
2. Period of embryo 2–8 wks of i.u. age
3. Period of fetus after 8 wks till birth.

◎ What are the different methods of studying growth?

These are:

Longitudinal studies = i.e. a specific set of subjects is followed on a long term basis at a particular interval of time and records are obtained and compared.

Cross sectional studies = i.e. performed at the same time. Here, different sets of subjects at different age group are collected, records are obtained and compared with each other.

◎ What is the role of vital staining in studying growth?

It gets deposited in the sites of rapidly growing bone. Alizarine red S stain as found in *madder plants*; tetracycline and trypon blue are some of the stains used. The major disadvantage of this method is that the animal has to be killed for results.

◎ How are the implants used as a method of studying the growth?

The implants are placed at particular sites in maxillary and mandibular bones. The subject is followed on a longitudinal basis by taking the lateral cephalograms at particular age of the subjects and studied. The position of implants does not change with growth and they are used for superimposing the serial cephalograms.

◎ Various sites of implant placement in maxilla are?

1. Hard palate behind maxillary deciduous canines.
2. Below ANS
3. Zygomatic process of maxilla.
4. Border b/w hard palate and alveolar process medial to first molars.

◎ Which are the various sites of implant placement in mandible?

1. In midline at the anterior aspect of symphysis.
2. 2 pins on RHS of the body of mandible below first premolar; and below and b/w 2nd premolar and the 1st molars.
3. 1 pin on the RHS ramus at the level of occlusal plane (OP). This becomes free in the soft tissues as growth occurs due to resorption of anterior border of the ramus.

◎ When does the Midsagittal suture close?

It does not close until the middle of 3rd decade of life.

◎ What is the relation of age and the growth / size of cranial base?

When related to the age, the size of the cranial base at

1. Birth is 55-60% of adult size;
2. 4-7 years is 94% of adult size; and
3. 8-13 years is 98% of adult size.

◎ What are the 2 methods of bone formation?

These are intramembranous and endochondral ossification.

◎ How does the ratio of the size of face vary with that of whole body with age?

When related to the age, the size of the face at Birth is 50 % of the size of the body; at 4–7 yrs is 33 % and at 8–13 yrs is 12 % i.e. 1:8 of the body size.

◎ Which all bones are intramembranous in development?

1. Pure intramembranous : Frontal, zygomatic, parietal, palatal, maxilla, vomer, nasal, lacrimal
2. Pure endochondral : Ethmoid, Inferior nasal concha
3. Mixed : Mandible, occipital, sphenoid, temporal

◎ What do you mean by the cephalocaudal gradient of growth?

Cephalocaudal gradient of growth means that the amount of growth of structures away from the head increases towards the caudal ends. For example, lower limbs grow more than the upper limbs; the mandible grows more and up to later age than maxilla.

It helps **decrease the overjet** which is especially marked during first 6 months of life. Mandible seems to erupt from below the cranium.

In newborn, the cranium is 8-9 x larger than face, an example of the cephalocaudal gradient of growth. Later on, the facial growth catches up.

◎ What is the general direction of growth of face with respect to skull and cranial base?

Downwards and Forwards.

◎ From which pharyngeal arch, the maxilla and mandible are formed?

First arch, i.e. mandibular arch gives rise to maxilla and mandible; Meckel's cartilage; malleus, incus, muscles of mastication and the anterior digastric m.

◎ How is the palate formed?

Palatal shelves arise from the maxillary processes. They first go vertically and then move horizontally with the lowered position of the tongue; then they fuse anteriorly with the primary palate (which arises from the median nasal process) and with one another. The fusion starts in the middle of the processes and proceeds anteriorly and posteriorly.

◎ How does the growth in maxillary Length occurs?

By apposition at maxillary tuberosity

◎ What do you mean by differential growth pattern?

Different tissues grow at Different rates at Different times. **Scammon's growth curves** show that lymphoid, nervous, somatic and genital tissues grow at different ages and rates. According to Scammon's growth studies, the Lymphoid > Neural > General > Genital tissues growth.

Neural tissue is of adult size at = 6–7 yrs age.

Lymphoid tissue is 200 % size at = late childhood phase; it starts involuting itself and becomes of normal size by 18 yrs age.

Genital tissues = grow at puberty; after it growth ceases. The start of menstruation in females and development of secondary sexual features in females is the sign of completion of growth in females. It starts increasing when the lymphoid tissues start decreasing at approx. 10 – 12 yrs of age.

◎ How does the growth of general tissues relate with time?

Rapid growth occurs = up to 2–3 yrs age.

Slow growth = 3–10 yrs age

Rapid growth = after 10 yrs to 18–20 yrs age.

◎ How does the development of face and neck region differ from other body parts?

Nearly all tissues of face and neck originate from ECTODERM (including muscles and bone also, which elsewhere in the body originate from the MESODERM). Most of these tissues develop from NCC. Most of facial structures arise from NCC - interference with their movement leads to deformities, e.g. Hemifacial microsomia, Mandibulofacial dysostosis, i.e. Treacher Collins synd - both U/L jaws involved especially lateral face is involved due to excessive cell death in trigeminal ganglion which affects NCCs (**N**eural **C**rest **C**ells).

◎ **Which is the most critical phase of the facial development?**

Most of the problems, which result in craniofacial anomalies arise in 3rd stage of development, i.e. 19-28 days (4th week). It is the period in which the clefts develop.

◎ **Which is the most common congenital defect of face?**

CLP. **Clefts arise during 4th developmental stage (first trimester).**

◎ **Which is the most common congenital defect of the body?**

Club foot

◎ **Tell us a few points about the development of palate?**

Formation of primary - palate is evident by 28-38 i.u. days; and of **secondary palate by 42-55 days i.u.** The primary palate develops from the frontonasal process, while the secondary palate develops from the palatal shelves from the maxillary process. Fusion of the shelves progresses from A to P and reaches the soft palate.

◎ **What are the derivatives of primary palate?**

It develops in the premaxilla and the alveolar process underlying it and part of the inside of the upper lip.

◎ **Which processes are involved in palatal development?**

- Maxillary process
- Palatal process from maxillary process
- Frontonasal process = forms the premaxillary region
- It develops during 8–12 wks of i.u life.

- Initial contact of palatal processes is in the central region of the palatal shelves.
- Ossification starts at 8th wk i.u. life.
- Midpalatal suture ossifies by 12–14 yrs of age.

◎ **How does the maturation of oral function progresses?**

It follows **a gradient from Anterior to Posterior**, for example

Speech	First sounds = bilabial	m, p, b
(A→P)	Tongue tip consonants	t, d
	Sibilants	s, z
	Posterior tongue positioning	r

◎ **When does the maxillary sinus develop.**

It develops at around 3rd month of life.

◎ **When can you see the MANDIBLE developing in the embryo?**

Ans: Mandible is recognizable in **shape at 8th week.**

◎ **What is the role of Meckle's cartilage during the mandibular development?**

Although Meckle's C is a cartilaginous structure, still the development of mandible is mainly intramembranous, with only small part is endochondral. Meckle's C acts as a splint, around which the bone of mandible develops and the cartilage itself does not take any part in the bone formation.

◎ **Which areas develop by endochondral ossification in mandible?**

Only 3 areas are endochondral in mandible, e. condyle, coronoid and mental areas.

◎ **What is the difference in the growth pattern of cranial base and cranial vault?**

Cranial base (neurocranium) grows especially at synchondroses; Cranial vault (desmocranium) grows by sutural growth. CRANIAL

BASE is endochondral especially of midline structures. Desmocranium = has neurocranial capsule and orofacial capsule.

◎ What are the remnants of Meckle's cartilage?

These are malleus, incus, mental ossicles, spine of sphenoid bone, anterior ligament of malleus and sphenomandibular ligament.

◎ Which is the first structure to develop in the primordium of lower jaw?

It is mandibular division of 5th N.

◎ How does the growth of neurocranium and splanchnocranium differ?

Neurocranium = follows neural growth pattern; Splanchnocranium (lower face) follows general / bodily growth pattern.

◎ What is the difference between the growth of bone and cartilage?

Cartilage grows both by INTERSTITIAL and APPOSITIONAL GROWTH. Bone grows by additive or apposition only (it can't grow by interstitial or expansile activity).

◎ How does the condylar cartilage differ from the epiphyseal cartilage?

Epiphyseal C (if transplanted) can grow independently - so it is **a primary cartilage** with genetic potential. But **condylar cartilage is secondary cartilage** and can not grow after transplantation.

◎ What is the difference of condylar cartilage with other hyaline cartilage of the body?

The condylar cartilage is a fibrocartilage; it has distinct collagen fibers and is affected by the environmental factors also during growth. The hyaline cartilage of the condyle is covered by a dense and thick fibrous connective tissue layer. Thus it not only increases by the interstitial growth, but also by the increase in thickness by the appositional growth beneath the connective tissues covering it.

Other hyaline cartilages of the body have indistinct collagen fibers and growth is affected by the epigenetic factors.

◎ **Where lies the biologic center of the growth of the face?**

Stationary biologic center lies in the body of sphenoid bone. It is marked in the cephalogram by the position of **foramen rotundum**.

◎ **Mandible develops by how many ossification centres?**

There is single ossification center for the development of mandible. It appears in 6th week i.u. life. It is present in the future premolar region, i.e. at the bifurcation of inferior alveolar n. in the mental and incisive branches. The ossification stops at the future mandibular lingula.

◎ **How does the growth of face and skull depend on functional matrices?**

Up to 5th year, it is Neurocranial dominance. After 5 year is the orofacial dominance of growth.

◎ **How are the Epigenetic factors different from the genetic factors?**

Epigenetic factors are genetically determined but influence in an indirect way by intermediary action on associated structures (eye, brain, etc.)

◎ **What is the influence of Nasal septum on the growth of maxilla?**

It is more important in Anteroposterior growth than vertical growth of maxilla.

◎ **What are synchondroses? Which synchondrosis affects the growth of the cranial base?**

Synchondroses are the sites of growth containing the intervening cartilage in between the two parts of the growing bone. So the growth is cartilagineous here. There are 4 main synchondroses affecting the growth of cranial base specifically and the facial skeleton generally. These are

- Sphenoethmoidal = close at 5-25 year (exactly unknown).
- Intersphenoidal = close at Birth.
- Sphenooccipital = close at 20th year = main synchondroses and **most important.**
- Inter occipital = close at 3-5 years.

• Which type of skeletal jaw malocclusion is seen in achondroplasia?

Skeletal class III relationship is present in this condition due to maxillary hypoplasia. It occurs due to absence of cartilagineous parts in the synchondroses of cranial base and hence the growth of cranial base is deficient. Since maxillary growth is affected by the growth of cranial base, so the maxillary AP deficiency is there.

◎ What is the position of Metopic suture?

It lies between the 2 halves of frontal bones before their fusion.

◎ What is the Direction of growth of the different craniosacral components?

a. Basal cranium = U/F

b. Maxilla = D/F

c. Mandible's condyle = U/B

d. Mandible = D/F

◎ What is the direction of mandibular rotation in horizontal and vertical growth patterns?

Mandible rotates in upward and forward direction in horizontal growth pattern leading to skeletal deep bite; while in downward and backward direction in vertical growth pattern leading to skeletal open bite.

◎ What is the direction of condylar growth in horizontal and vertical growth patterns?

It is upward and forward in horizontal growth pattern; and upward and backward in vertical growth pattern.

◎ How does the Growth of maxilla occur?

Maxilla is mainly **INTRAMEMBRANOUS** except;

- Paranasal processes of nasal capsule
- Alveolar border of zygomatic process

2 areas: (1) Neural and alveolar areas; (2) Frontal, zygomatic, palatal processes.

A passive / **secondary displacement** of nasomaxillary complex is D and F due to cranial base growth.

Primary displacement of nasomaxillary complex occurs by growth of maxillary tuberosity in posterior direction.

◎ Where lie the ossification centers of the maxilla?

3 primary ossification centers = one above canine fossa for maxilla proper and two for premaxilla.

◎ What is the prenatal growth of maxilla?

It arises from a single center of ossification into 2 areas based on the relation to the infraorbital nerve. These are neural and alveolar areas; and frontal, zygomatic and palatal processes.

Maxilla is an intramembranous bone except the paranasal processes of the nasal capsule and the cartilaginous areas at the alveolar border of the zygomatic process.

◎ How do the craniomaxillary sutures affect the growth of maxilla?

Main sutures are frontonasal, frontomaxillary, zygomaticomaxillary, zygomaticotemporal, and pterygopalatine. All are oblique and parallel to each other; growth there moves the maxilla D/F or cranium U/B. But sutural growth is secondary.

◎ Which is the Basic maxillary skeletal unit?

Infraorbital neurovascular triad

◎ Which are the general features of maxillary growth?

a. Maxillary width is completed quite at early age, (i.e. follows neural growth curve - as it is attached to cranial base.

b. Elongation of dental arches occurs at free (distal) ends only.

Actual changes, which occur in maxilla, are controlled by EPIGENETIC FACTORS. Indirect genetic control is known as EPIGENETIC.

c. Growth completion sequence in dimensions with age = WDH (width earliest completed).

d. The position of maxilla is dependent on the growth at the sphenooccipital and sphenoethmoidal synchondroses.

e. While growth of cranial base is mostly endochondral, the growth of cranial vault and maxilla is intramembranous.

f. Early midface horizontal growth is tied to endochondrally induced anterior cranial base increase.

g. In late stages = vertical growth dominates the horizontal growth in maxilla.

h. Mainly sutural and remodelling–Translation and transformation.

i. Midpalatal suture: does not start closing till 8–10 yrs of age.

j. Nasal septum shows endochondral growth.

◎ **How does the nasomaxillary complex grow in the face?**

It is due to growth at sutures, surface remodelling, and displacement. Nasal cartilage also plays its role in its growth. A deficiency in nasal C for example, due to trauma, leads to a deficient maxilla.

◎ **What is the Meckel's cartilage?**

It acts only as a Template for **intramembranous** growth of mandible and does not contribute to mandible bone, which develops lateral to Meckel's cartilage. It is the cartilage of first pharyngeal arch.

◎ **How does the ossification of mandible occur?**

It ossifies by **2 ossification centres,** one each in the area of future mental foramen, (appear in 6 week I.U.) lateral to Meckel's cartilage, **Ossification stops at a point, which later becomes LINGULA.**

◎ **What are the remnants of Meckel's cartilage?**

These are malleus, incus, spine of sphenoid, sphenomandibular ligament, etc.

◎ **What are the general features of growth of MANDIBLE?**

a. It starts developing prenatally and is recognizable in shape by 8th week I.U.

b. Lower jaw is the **first to develop** in the facial skeleton.

c. Its growth **follows GENERAL TISSUE growth curve**, while that of vault follows neural growth curve.

d. Ratio of alveolar plate length to the total mandibular length is relatively constant. Also, the ratio of width b/w the mandibular angle to the total width is relatively constant during the fetal life.

e. **At birth** = Size of mandibular arch is sufficient to accommodate all primary teeth if erupted.

f. 2 halves of mandible fuse by 16-18 months age.

g. Main growth of mandible after birth occurs at condyle, Ramus, Alveolar bone

h. D/F movement of mandible is primarily *passive translation.*

i. Mandibular growth is considered more of an **adaptive shift**.

j. **Active transformation** = minor D/F changes but mainly U/B compensatory growth of ramus.

k. Mandibular growth is more sustained in boys than in girls (i.e. up to 25 years age). Distance between mental foramina = changes little after 6 years age (i.e. width of mandible).

l. **Mental foramen** level changes with growth, from near mandibular border (infants) to middle of the body (in adults) to at alveolar crest (in edentulous patient).

m. Level of **mandibular foramen** lies below OP in children and at the level of OP in adults.

◎ Describe CONDYLE as the growth site of mandible?

Condyle is the major growth CENTRE of mandible, it has **fibrocartilage,** which is a secondary cartilage, grows by proliferation of cartilage. **Condyle is the only bone in body** which shows ***both interstitial and appositional growth.*** Peak of condylar growth is at 12–14 yrs age and it ceases at around 20 yrs age.

Condyle grows in U and B direction - so mandible moves in D and F direction, along an arc, which runs from foramen ovale to mandibular foramen to mental foramen (**unloaded nerve concept**).

Condyles are not the primary site of mandibular growth, but are loci with secondary, compensatory growth potential.

◎ What do you mean by basal tubular part?

It protects mandibular nerve (**unloaded nerve concept**) and follows a logarithmic spiral in its D/F growth.

◎ What is the most constant portion of mandible?

It is the ARC from F. ovale to mandibular foramen to mental foramen.

◎ What structures are the functional matrices for the growth of alveolar bone?

Teeth are the main factors for the growth of alveolar bones. In a place where the tooth is congenitally missing, the bone is deficient. That is why, the enucleation of first premolar and 3rd molars tooth buds is not considered during the orthodontic treatment, till at least half of root development occurs.

◎ Describe growth of CHIN?

Only human and elephant have got chin.

Area of chin just above symphysis menti is resorptive, which gives the chin its prominence. The area at the pogonion is depository.

◎ Describe the RAMAL GROWTH?

In infancy = the ramus is located at approx. primary first molar area.

Growth occurs along the **V-principle**. Anterior border is resorptive to provide space for eruption of permanent molars.

After **6 years age**, greatest increase in size of mandible occurs distal to first molars.

Posterior surface is depository.

Ramal growth **provides space vertically** in which both U/L alveolar bones grow, the teeth being their functional matrices.

◎ What is the concept of LATE MANDIBULAR GROWTH?

Occurs in horizontal direction and is mainly responsible for lower anterior crowding, rather than mandibular third molars, which appears, develops or increases in the adult age / post-pubertal age (20–30 years age).

(L) incisors tend to upright under the terminal horizontal growth increments, which occurs due to **U and F rotation of mandible**, leading to lingual movement of lower incisors and their crowding.

◎ What is the difference in growth patterns of CRANIUM and the face?

Cranium growth occurs in **DW (H)** i.e. growth in D is most rapid, with growth in W and H in that order. In **FACE, the pattern is HD (W), i. e.** H shows greatest incremental changes with age and W shows least incremental change with age. So **at birth, height of cranium and width of face are closest to adult size.**

◎ What is the generally sequence of growth completion?

Growth is generally completed first in head, then in W of face and last in L (D) of face.

◎ What is the difference in the velocity of growth of cranium and the face?

In cranium, the D>W>H; and in face there is H>D>W, i.e. at birth, the H of cranium and W of the face are the closest to the adult size.

◎ How does the growth in female differ from the males?

Female pubertal spurt occurs 2-3 yrs ahead of that of male. Also, there are only 2 spurts in females while males generally show 3 spurts. Females mature earlier than males.

THEORIES OF GROWTH

◎ Which are the theories of growth?

1. Genetic
2. Sutural theory by Sicher
3. Cartilaginous theory by Scott
4. Functional matrix theory by Moss
5. von Limborgh's theory
6. Enlow's expanding V principle
7. Enlow's counterpart principle

◎ Which is the most important theory of growth?

It is the **functional matrix theory by Moss.** It is based on the functional cranial component theory of van der Klaauw.

FCC

Functional matrix

- Periosteal matrix
- Capsular matrix
  1. Neurocranial capsule
  2. Orofacial capsule

skeletal unit

1. Macroskeletal unit
2. Microskeletal unit

◎ Which are the 2 main functional matrices?

These are periosteal matrix and capsular matrix.

◎ Which are the main theories of growth?

There are 3 main theories, i.e. Sicher's sutural theory; Scott's cartilagineous theory; Moss's functional matrix theory.

◎ **What is the idea behind functional matrix theory of growth?**

It emphasizes that the osseous growth of the skull is entirely secondary. There is dominance of non-osseous structures of the craniofacial complex over the bony parts.

◎ **Which factors affect the growth as given by Von Limborgh?**

1. Intrinsic genetic
2. Local epigenetic
3. General epigenetic
4. Local environmental
5. General environmental factors

◎ **What is the Major difference in various growth theories?**

It is the LOCATION at which genetic control is expressed.

◎ **What is the difference b/w the growth SITE and the growth center?**

Site is a location where growth occurs; **CENTER** is a location **at which independent, genetically controlled growth occurs,** i.e. independent of environment.

◎ **Which are the 2 capsular matrices affecting the growth of face?**

They are neurocranial and orofacial capsules.

◎ **What is a GROWTH SPURT?**

The growth never occurs with uniformity. There are periods when there is an increase in growth. These are ka growth spurts.

	Female	**Male**
First peak (childhood)	3 years	3 years
2nd peak (Juvenile)	6-7 years	7-9 years
3rd peak (Prepubertal)	11-12 years	14-15 years

◎ What are the main features of the growth spurts?

a. More boys to have 2-3 peaks.

b. Girls show only 2 peaks.

c. Very few girls show mixed dentition period growth spurt, but all show pubertal growth spurt.

d. So mixed dentition jaw changes (with functional appliances) is more successful in boys.

e. Females mature earlier (2-3 years) than males, so early treatment is more critical in girls than in boys.

f. During pubertal growth period = there is directional change from vertical to horizontal.

g. Growth modulation therapy is better and results are stable, if given during the spurts period.

◎ What are Tweed's growth trends?

Based on the angles FMA, IMPA, FMIA, Tweed described growth trends in type A, B ,C.

1. Type A = maxilla and mandible grow D and F in unison. It is seen by no changes in the ANB angle; 25% of patients are in this category.
2. Type B = here, entire growth D and F, but the maxilla grows more rapidly than the mandible, and so ANB angle increases, 15% patients belong to this category.
3. Type C = mandible grows rather D and F at a faster rate as compared to maxilla, it shows the decrease in ANB. 60% patients, i.e. largest amount of patients are in this category.

◎ What are the periods of growth and dental development according to Hellman?

1. Stage I = is the period of early infancy before the completion of the deciduous dentition.
2. Stage II = it is the period of late infancy at the completion of the deciduous dentition.

3. Stage III = is the period of childhood when the permanent first molars are erupting or have taken their positions.
4. Sage IV = is the period of pubescence when the second molars are erupting or have taken their positions.
5. Stage V = is the period of adulthood when the 3rd molars are erupting or have taken their place.
6. Stage VI = is the period of old age when the occlusal surfaces of molars are worn off to the extent of obliterating the pattern of the grooves.
7. Stage VII = designates the period of senility.

Self-Assessment Questions

1. What are various clinical implications of growth?
2. What do you mean by SAFETY-VALVE mechanism?
3. What is the UGLY-DUCKLING STAGE?
4. What is meant by BIPHASIC R_x?
5. What are different components of functional matrix?
6. What is the difference between primary and secondary displacement of growth?
7. What all are different fontanelles in the skull of an infant and which is the largest one?
8. What is the role of fontanelles?

Reader's Notes

3

Clinical Implications

◎ Which are the various self correcting malocclusion conditions?

Certain conditions, which look abnormal during their existence but are normal for that age and are the developmental indicators are called as self-correcting anomalies. These get corrected as the child grows. For example, open bite in the gum pads; spaced primary dentition, deep bite, flush terminal plane, ugly duckling stage, attrition of primary teeth, edge to edge bite, retrognathic mandible at birth and early age, digit sucking habit till 3–4 yrs age, etc.

◎ How does the growth help us in orthodontic treatment?

The treatment is fast and results are stable. Functional appliances to bring the mandible forward are more favorable in growth phase especially during the spurts and give orthopedic effects. The best age for functional appliance treatment is approx. 10 yrs in females and 12 yrs in males.

Also, maxilla can be moved forward best during 8–9 yrs age to treat maxillary hypoplasia / retrognathism to bring a stable, orthopedic effect.

◎ How does the intercanine width change with growth?

	Maxilla	Mandibular
M	18 years	9-10 years
F	12 years	9-10 years

Intercanine width increases more in spaced dentition, more in maxilla, and up to a later age in maxilla.

◎ What is the safety valve mechanism?

Maxillary intercanine width acts as **SAFETY VALVE**, i.e. when the final horizontal growth of mandible occurs especially in males, it causes a forward movement of mandibular base with teeth.

In both sexes, the maxillary intercanine dimension serves as a safety valve for pubertal growth spurt, where basal horizontal mandibular growth is partly unmatched by maxilla, as mandible grows D and F.

◎ What are the advantages of early orthodontic treatment?

These are the possibility of growth modifications, prevention and interception of the abnormal conditions, advantage of growth during treatment, improving the psychological status of the child, and a better cooperation of the child during that age. For example, the cross bite, especially anterior cross bite should be corrected as soon as possible, as it may lead to skeletal class III mandible if left unattended, due to unrestricted mandibular growth.

◎ Can we do surgical intervention during the growth phase for the severe skeletal discrepancy?

It is not indicated especially for mandible, since there are extreme chances of attaining the same skeletal condition after some time due to ensuing mandibular growth on the same abnormal pattern. The surgery is to be done only after the completion or slowing down of the growth, i.e. after approx. 18 yrs of age. The results can be considered stable after that age.

◎ Does the tooth movement depend on the age of the patient?

The tooth movement is faster and easier to start in the children as the bones are pliable, less dense, and softer, there is more growth component in children, apical foramen of the teeth are wider and so there are less chances of devitalisation of the teeth under same amount of forces as used for the adult patients. Also all kinds of the tooth movements cannot be done in adults as it largely depends on their periodontal condition also.

◎ What precaution must be taken during the orthodontic treatment of an adult patient?

You should use very light forces during treatment as the apical foramen are narrow and so forces might cause the occlusion of blood vessels at the apices of the teeth leading to loss of vitality. Also, tipping should be avoided in these patient.

◎ Is the intrusion of any advantage in patient having bone loss and periodontal pockets?

Yes. It has been observed that the intrusion causes the decrease in the depth of the periodontal pockets and helps in the increase of the relative alveolar bone height.

◎ How does the growth in female differ to that in males?

The growth in females is generally completed 2–3 yrs before males.

◎ What is indicated by the onset of menstruation in females?

It shows that growth spurt is nearly completed.

◎ What are the GROWTH COMPLETION sequences?

1. W = Both jaws + arches = before adolescent growth spurt especially on canine regions, but in M2 / M3 region, width increases due to jaws growth in the length posteriorly.
2. D (Length) = continues through period of puberty.

   Female = 14-15 years (2-3 years after menstruation).

   Male = approx. 18 years (4 years after sexual maturity).
3. H in Females = 17-18 years and in Males = early 20's

Reader's Notes

4

Development of Dentition

◎ What are Gum pads?

Are the alveolar processes at the time of birth.

Dental arches of an infant till no teeth erupted are ka gum pads.

Touch in future primary first molar region only.

Anterior open bite is present which helps in tongue positioning during suckling.

Anterior overjet is due to smaller lower jaw.

Posterior overjet due to wider upper arch than lower.

◎ When is the intercuspation of occlusal height in primary dentition established for the first time?

At eruption of primary first molars only.

Deep bite in primary dentition is due to more upright incisors.

◎ What are the natal and neonatal teeth?

Natal teeth are present at the time of birth; while the neonatal teeth erupt during the first month of age.

◎ What is the force of tooth eruption?

Eruption force of tooth is = b/w 2–10 gms in the pre-functional phase.

◎ What is the pressure of the eruption of the tooth?

Pressure of eruption = 0.2 gm / mm^2 of the enface root surface, as according to Ricketts.

◎ In which units, the rate of dental eruption is measured?

Rate of tooth eruption is measured in = microns / hr units.

◎ What is the latest concept of dental eruption?

Latest theory of eruption is that the eruptive forces are generated in PDL rather than at the root apex.

◎ What is the Baume's classification of occlusion in primary dentition?

Flush terminal plane	76% (to be observed most critically)
Mesial step	14%
Distal step	10%

- Distal step =

  (a) change to Class II, if minimum growth differential is there.

  (b) change in end–on, by loss of lee way space and forward mandibular growth.

- FTP =

  (a) change to end- on if minimum growth differential is there.

  (b) change in Class I due to loss of leeway space of mandibular E

  (c) change in Class II if maxillary E is lost before mandibular E.

- Mesial step =

  (a) change to Class I if minimun growth differential is there.

  (b) change to Class III, due to loss of leeway space and forward mandibular growth.

◎ What is the flush terminal plane (FTP) relationship?

When the distal surfaces of upper and lower primary second molars are in the same plane, it is ka FTP.

In mesial step, distal surface of lower second molar is mesial to that of upper second molar.

In distal step, distal surface of lower second molar is distal to that of upper second molar.

◎ What is meant by an open dentition and a closed dentition?

Developmental spacing in deciduous dentition, if present, it is known as **open dentition.** If absent, it is known as **closed dentition.**

Given below in the table are the possibility of crowding in the Permanent Dentition depending on the crowding present in the deciduous dentition.

Class	In deciduous teeth	Crowding chances in permanent teeth
I	Crowded	10 in 10
II	No spaces	7 in 10
III	≤ 3 mm spacing	5 in 10
IV	3–6 mm spacing	2 in 10
V	> 6 mm spacing	None

◎ What is the Primary spacing / physiological /developmental spacing?

It is present in the primary dentition. It is the normal developmental sequence; and is an important requirement for proper development of dentition; occurs due to growth, helps in proper alignment of bigger sized permanent teeth; occurs 70% in maxilla and 63% in mandible.

◎ What is the sequence of eruption of primary teeth?

It is ABDCE. Primary teeth start developing at 6th wk of i.u life; first primary tooth erupts at approx. 6 mos. of age; and by 2½–3 yrs age, all primary teeth are present in the oral cavity.

◎ What do you mean by Primate/simian/anthropoid spaces?

These are found mesial to primary maxillary canines and distal to primary mandibular canines; named so as it is found in primates, i.e. between BC/ CD.

◎ Why there is deep bite in the primary dentition?

It is due to more upright primary incisors. The intrinsical angle is approx. 170 degrees as compared to 131 degrees in permanent dentition. It decreases due to attrition of primary incisors, eruption of molars and by forward mandibular growth.

Bite depth in Permanent Dentition is less than in primary dentition. It is due to decreased intrinsical angle, due to forward eruption of permanent incisors. Also they are not that upright on their basal bone.

◎ What do you mean by Mixed Dentition Period (MDP)?

It is the period of dentition when a few primary and permanent teeth are present in the mouth. It begins with the eruption of first permanent molars at 6 yeas of age, generally in end-on relationship, marks the Stage I of natural bite opening.

◎ What is the natural bite opening?

It is the decrease in the overbite due to eruption of the permanent molars in the oral cavity. It occurs 3 times in the life of an individual, i.e. at the time of eruption of 1st, 2nd and 3rd permanent molars. So the permanent molars are called as natural bite openers.

◎ What is mechanism of natural bite opening?

When the molars erupt, the soft tissues overlying the molars is swollen and it comes in contact when in mastication or swallowing causes pain. So the patients learn to keep the contact away from it. It causes a gap in the area anterior to molar region and gives time for the supra-eruption of the teeth.

◎ What is meant by First transitional period / early Mixed Dentition Period (MDP)?

It starts with the eruption of 6,1,2 teeth; mostly lower teeth erupt first at 6-8 years age. Here, we can see the 3 relations of permanent first molars, viz. Mesial step, distal step and flush terminal plane (FTP) relation.

Correction of FTP/end-on relation to class I occurs by utilization of physiologic space, leeway space and differential forward growth of the mandible.

◎ **What is meant by Early mesial shift?**

It occurs in **open dentition at 6-7 years age**, due to closure of primate spaces by pressure of erupting permanent molars.

◎ **What do you mean by Late mesial shift?**

It occurs **in closed dentition at 10-11 years** age, due to closure of leeway spaces after shedding of primary second molars.

◎ **What is Incisal liability?**

It is the difference between sizes of primary and permanent incisors; it is 7.6 mm in upper and 6.0 mm in lower arch. It is overcome by– utilization of physiological interdental spacing, incisor inclination labially, and increased intercanine width **(Warren Mayne's principles).**

METHOD	MAXILLA	MANDIBLE
I/D spacing	0 –10 mm, av. = 4 mm	0–6 mm, av. = 3 mm
Increase in intercanine width	4.5 mm	3 mm
Incisor position	2.2 mm	1.3 mm

Incisor liability: Difference in size of permanent and primary teeth, the space comes from 3 sources:

1. *Increase in intercanine width* = 2 mm, M>F, U>L

   Girls have greater liability to incisor crowding.

2. *Labial positioning* of permanent incisors = 1-2 mm

3. *Repositioning* of mandibular canines distally in primate spaces when mandibular LIs erupt = 1 mm space. (But not in (U) arch, as primate space is between B and C there.

◎ Why a class III relationship is very rare in primary dentition period?

In primary dentition, An equivalent of Class III is never seen, due to growth pattern of mandible, which lags behind the maxilla.

Also C2 D2 is not seen in primary dentition.

◎ How much mesial movement of the permanent first molar is required for attaining class I relation from the FTP?

Approx. 3.5 mm of movement of mandibular first molar forward with respect to maxillary first molar is required for smooth transition to class I relation in permanent dentition (i.e. a one half cusp transition in molar relation).

◎ What is Inter-transitional period?

It is a quite period, at 8 —10 years of age; here no change is seen in dentition. No teeth erupt during this time period.

◎ What is Late mixed dentition / second transitional period?

It is the period of dentition in the age of 10–12 yrs when there is eruption of 3,4,5; Transition in chewing pattern develops in conjunction with eruption of permanent canines at age 12 years.

◎ What is leeway space of Nance?

It is the difference between MD sizes of CDE and 3,4,5; it is 1.8 mm in maxilla and 3.4 mm in mandible; it is mostly due to primary mandibular second molar size ka E–space (2–3 mm), helps in late mesial shift to achieve class I molars.

◎ What is E-space?

It is the space provided by the primary mandibular second molar when the second premolar erupts after its shedding. It is approx 3 mm.

◎ What is Space age?

It is the mixed dentition period (MDP). This is the most important phase of dentition development and should be very critically observed.

◎ Why the attrition is considered important in the primary dentition and Mixed Dentition Period?

Pronounced attrition in MDP is observed to help in–decrease in deep bite, prevent interlocking of the cusps by flattening them and thus paving way for unhindered forward growth of mandible.

◎ How does the Deep bite decreases during transition of dentition?

It occurs by eruption of permanent molars, attrition of incisors and forward movement of mandible due to growth.

Intercanine width increases more in spaced dentition, more in maxilla, up to a later age in maxilla.

◎ What is meant by Secondary spacing?

It occurs in closed dentition with eruption of lower incisors, which pushes primary mandibular canine laterally. It creates space for proper eruption of maxillary lateral incisors. It helps to increase the intercanine width in both arches and increase in arch circumference in maxilla.

◎ What do you mean by tertiary spacing?

It is the spacing created due to extraction etc.

◎ What is Ugly duckling stage of Broadbent?

In maxillary arch, at 8-9 years age, canines press the roots of laterals and so root crowding occurs, crowns move distally, spaces develop b/w crowns of incisors. It should not be disturbed till eruption of canines, as it is a self-correcting anomaly.

◎ How does the Arch length change from Mixed Dentition Period (MDP) to the Permanent Dentition Period (PDP)?

It decreases by 2–3 mm when MDP changes to PDP, both from anterior and posterior sides. The anteriors erupt in upright situation and with growth of mandible. Also posterior teeth move mesially throughout life due to attrition, loss of leeway space and anterior component of force of occlusion.

Also the arch width does not increase b/w 2 ½–6 years of age; and the arch perimeter does not increase b/w 2 ½–6 years of age.

◎ **When is the largest arch length available in the dentition?**

It is before eruption of first permanent molar.

◎ **What are the signs of incipient malocclusion?**

These are–lack of interdental spacing in primary dentition, crowding in permanent incisors in MDP and premature loss of primary canines especially mandibular due to the eruption of lateral incisors which cause root resorption of canines if arch length is deficient in the mandibular arch.

◎ **Which are the self-correcting anomalies?**

GUM PADS STAGE	PRIMARY D P	MIXED D P
Open bite	Deep bite	End-on molars
Increased overjet	FTP	Ugly-duckling stage
Tongue in between gum pads	Primary spacing	< 2 mm of lower incisors crowding
	Primate spacing	
	Small mandible	
	More upright incisors	

◎ **How does the chewing pattern of child differ from that of an adult?**

The adults open the mouth straight and then moves it laterally during chewing, while the child moves laterally.

◎ **What are various features of development of dentition?**

1. **Natural bite opening** – at 6, 12, 18 years of age, with eruption of permanent molars.
2. 3 periods of bite opening (Schwarz)
3. 6 years =when First molar erupts, 12 years = 2nd molar molar erupts, 18 years = 3rd molar erupts.

4. U/L permanent incisors erupt lingual to primary teeth and move forward under the tongue pressure as they erupt.
5. 7-8 years age = critical period
6. Sudden change during the eruption of the CI and LI is shown by = **1.5 mm crowding** in both M and F. Average female recovers slightly better than males.
7. No great relief of crowding in incisor region is expected after full eruption of L.I.
8. Most crowding = (L) anterior segments
9. Occlusal contact is only 2-6% in 24 hours period.
10. Primary incisors are more vertical and interincisal angle is greater causing deep bite.

- Mandibular CI, LI seem to erupt from LINGUAL
- Maxillary L.I. = no labial gingival bulge.
- Maxillary second molar erupts D and F
- Maxillary third molar erupts D and B and outward

◎ How does the apical inclinations of upper and lower teeth differ?

Axial inclination of maxillary teeth tend to converge apically especially at the end of the arch and mandibular axes tend to diverge following the Curve of Spee. Crowns of maxillary posterior teeth and canines and of all mandibular teeth are lingually inclined, (labial root torque), whole of maxillary incisors are labially inclined (i.e. labial crown torque).

Self Assessment Questions

1. What are different types of crowdings?
2. What is the eruption sequence of primary and permanent teeth?
3. What is the eruption age of various permanent teeth?
4. Define chronologic age, dental age and skeletal age? Which is most reliable?
5. What do you mean by self-correcting anomalies?

Reader's Notes

5

Stomatognathic System

◎ **How many muscles are attached at the mandible?**

13

◎ **What do you mean by isotonic and the isometric contraction of the muscle?**

In isotonic contraction, there is shortening of the muscle. In isometric contraction, the muscle contracts to resist an external force, without actual shortening of the muscle.

The greatest strength of the contractions is felt when the muscle approximates its resting length.

Maximum force of the muscle occurs when all the fibers are stimulated to fire.

◎ **What are the two types of swallowing patterns?**

The two types of swallowing patterns seen during the functional development are: infantile swallow and the adult / mature swallow.

◎ **How does the infantile swallowing differ from the mature / adult swallow?**

Main features of infantile swallowing pattern are

1. Jaws are separated. Teeth are apart.
2. Tongue is brought forward b/w the gum pads.
3. Mandible is stabilized by the facial muscles / 7th nerve muscles and the tongue.

4. Infantile swallow gradually disappears with the eruption of the buccal teeth in the primary dentition.

Main features of adult swallow are:

1. Tongue is contained with in the arches.
2. Teeth are together, i.e. in occlusion.
3. Jaws are stabilized by the 5th nerve muscles, i.e. mandibular elevators muscles.
4. Tip of the tongue is near the incisive papilla / rugae area of the palate, above and behind the incisors.
5. There is minimum contraction of lips during the mature swallow.

◎ **What do you mean by the transitional phase?**

The period of development during which infantile pattern changes to adult pattern. It occurs during 6–12 months of age.

◎ **At approx. what age, the infantile swallow changes to adult swallow?**

At approx. 18 mos. of age.

◎ **What are the phases of swallowing?**

According to Fletcher, 4 phases are: preparatory swallow; oral phase; pharyngeal phase and the esophageal phase.

◎ **What is the frequency of swallowing of an average individual?**

About once a minute b/w meals and approx. 9 times a minute during eating. An approx of 2400 somatic and visceral swallows occur during a 24-hr period.

◎ **What are the Benninghoff's lines or the trajectories of force?**

These are the natural lines of functional stresses in the bone.

◎ **What are the trajectories of maxilla?**

These are – the frontonasal buttress, malar-zygomatic buttress; and pterygoid buttress.

◎ **Which are the vertical pillars and horizontal reinforcing members of the maxilla?**

The vertical pillars are – canine pillar; zygomatic pillar and the pterygoid pillars,

The supra- and infraorbital bony eminences and the zygomatic buttresses are the horizontal reinforcers of the vertical pillars.

◎ **What are the trajectories of mandible?**

These are passing through:

1. Lower border of mandible
2. Mylohyoid ridge
3. Condyle to condyle along the symphysis.

The trabecular columns radiate from beneath the teeth in the alveolar process and join together in a common stress pillar that ends in the condyle.

◎ **What movements occur in the upper and lower compartment of the TMJ?**

Gliding in the upper and rotatory in the lower compartment.

◎ **What is the law of orthogonality or Wolff's law?**

Trabecular alignment of the bones is due primarily to functional forces (according to Wolff) is known as **Law of Orthogonality.**

◎ **What is the Law of Transformation of bone?**

It implies that the stresses of tension or pressure on bone stimulate the bone formation.

◎ **What is Buccinator mechanism?**

It involves Orbicularis oris m, Buccinator m and Superior constrictor m of pharynx; the later 2 muscles are attached at *pterygomandibular raphe*. It helps to guide the eruption of teeth in normal arch form by its moulding effect and keeps the pressure of tongue from inside balanced from outside. So the teeth erupt in that **neutral zone**. The total force of tongue is more than the buccal and cheek muscles, that difference is compensated by the forces of PDL.

◎ **What do you mean by Chondrocranium?**

It is a continuous plate of cartilage, extends from nasal capsule to foramen magnum. Most anterior part of chondrocranium is Nasal capsule.

◎ **Where lies the major center of growth of long bones?**

In epiphyseal plate cartilage which has uncalcified cartilage.

◎ **What is the normal position of tongue in newborn / infant?**

The tip occupies the space b/w the gum pads both during the postural resting position and during function.

◎ **Which is main muscle of tongue functioning during swallowing?**

It is genioglossus. It helps in plunger like, suckle swallowing.

◎ **What are the movements of hyoid bone during various mandibular movements?**

It moves D and B with opening of the mandible; U and F with the closure; and backwards with the retrusion of mandible.

◎ **What is Bennett movement?**

During the lateral shift of the mandible, the articular disc / the condyle moves towards the side of the working side. It is ka Bennett movement.

◎ **Which are the phases of the mastication?**

There are 6 phases of the mastication, viz

1. Preparatory phase
2. Food contact
3. Crushing phase
4. Tooth contact
5. Grinding phase
6. Centric occlusion.

Self Assessment Review

1. What do you mean by Adenoid facies?
2. How does Adenoid facies develop?
3. Which lymphoid group of tissues is involved as adenoids?
4. What are the different causes of mouth breathing?
5. What are different causes of arch narrowing?
6. What is buccinator mechanism?
7. What do you mean by NEUTRAL ZONE?
8. What do you understand by FREEWAY SPACE?

Reader's Notes

6

Occlusion

◎ For how much period, the teeth are in contact during a 24 hr period?

Only 2–6 % of the time in 24 -hr.

◎ What do you mean by normal and the ideal?

Normal is always a range in the physiology and anatomy; while the ideal is a rigidly set entity and so its very few examples are there in the nature.

◎ What is PREEMERGENT ERUPTION?

Eruptive movements begin soon after the roots begin to form - because metabolic activity in PDL plays a major role in eruption.

◎ What is POST-EMERGENT ERUPTION?

It occurs till the teeth come in occlusion after eruption in oral cavity and also to keep pace with occlusal attrition. Eruption occurs mainly at night.

◎ What is JUVENILE OCCLUSAL EQUILIBRIUM?

Teeth, which are in function, erupt at a rate, which parallels the rate of VERTICAL GROWTH of mandibular ramus.

◎ What do you mean by ideal occlusion?

It is just a theoretical concept which includes the idealized principles and the features that an occlusion should have.

◎ What do you mean by physiological occlusion?

It is the condition which deviates in one or more ways from the ideal but is still well adapted to its surroundings without pathological manifestations.

◎ What do you mean by balanced occlusion?

In it, the balanced and equal contacts are there b/w upper and lower teeth in the entire arch during all excursive movements. It is the concept mostly followed in complete denture fabrication for its stability.

◎ What do you mean by therapeutic occlusion?

An occlusion modified to change the non-physiologic occlusion to a physiological occlusion.

◎ What do you mean by functional occlusion?

It the working side contacts of the teeth which occur in the arch segment towards which the mandible moves.

◎ What do you mean by traumatic occlusion?

It is due to abnormal occlusal stresses which tends to produce or has produced the injury to the periodontium.

◎ What is a traumatogenic occlusion?

This is the term used which causes the trauma to the investing tissues due to abnormal occlusal stresses. So the term traumatic occlusion is a wrong misnomer of traumatogenic occlusion. It occurs due to loss of capability of the tissues to bear even the normal occlusal stresses.

◎ What do you mean by centric occlusion?

It is the maximum intercuspation of teeth when upper and lower jaws are brought together.

◎ What do you mean by eccentric occlusion?

Any deviation from the centric occlusion is ka eccentric occlusion. It includes the lateral and protrusive movements.

◎ **What is centric relation?**

It is the skeletal relation of maxilla and mandible in which the condyles are in their most superior and retruded position in the glenoid fossa with the articular disc properly interposed. It is aka terminal hinge position, i.e. THP.

◎ **What do you mean by malocclusion?**

An occlusal relation which is not normal is ka malocclusion.

◎ **What do you mean by group function occlusion?**

The occlusion in which posterior teeth of the working side contact with each other and disocclude the nonworking side.

◎ **What do you mean by canine protected occlusion?**

In it, the canines on the working side contact during the lateral movement and disocclude the non working side teeth. It is mostly seen in young and unworn dentition. It is the most preferred scheme of occlusion.

◎ **What do you mean by nonfunctional occlusion?**

These are the contacts occurring on the nonworking side during lateral movements. It is damaging to the tissues.

◎ **What do you mean by protrusive functional occlusion?**

It occurs when the mandible moves forward and slides along the lingual inclines of the maxillary anterior teeth and disocclude the posterior teeth.

◎ **What do you mean by centric holding cusps?**

These cusps are the main cusps which come in cusp to fossa relationship b/w upper and lower teeth. The facial cusps of mandibular and the palatal cusps of maxillary teeth are the central holding cusps. These are also called as supporting cusps or the stamp cusps.

◎ What do you mean by non-supporting cusps?

The maxillary buccal and the mandibular lingual cusps. They are also ka guiding cusps, as they help to guide the mandible during the excursive movements.

◎ What do you mean by curve of Spee?

If a line is drawn through the buccal cusps of lower posterior teeth till the canine tip, it takes a form of a curve in the AP direction. It is ka the curve of Spee.

◎ What do you mean by curve of Wilson?

It is the medio-lateral curve passing through the buccal and lingual cusp tips of mandibular posterior teeth. It is due to the inward inclination of the lower posterior teeth. It aligns the teeth parallel to the direction of medial pterygoid muscles action.

◎ What do you mean by curve of Monson?

Curves of spee and Wilson extended to all the posterior teeth.

◎ What are ANDREW'S 6 keys of normal occlusion?

These are

1. *Molar inter-arch relation*, i.e. MB cusp of upper first molar should lie in the MB groove of mandibular first molar. Also, the ML cusp of upper first molar should be lying in the central fossa of lower first molar. Distal marginal ridge of upper first molars occludes with mesial marginal ridge of lower second molar.
2. *Mesiodistal crown angulation* = i.e. tip.
3. *Labio-lingual crown inclination* = i.e. torque
4. *Absence of rotations*. The rotated posterior teeth take more space, while the rotated anterior teeth give the space.
5. *Tight contacts,* i.e. absence of spacing.
6. *Curve of Spee*.

INCIDENCE AND RECOGNITION OF THE MALOCCLUSION:

- Majority of malocclusions are the Class I m.o. (60%).
- Crowding is the major component of malocclusion characteristic.
- Shape of dental arch form goes with the form of the face.
- 75 % of arches are ellipse, 20 % are parabola and only 5 % are of U–/ square shape.
- Bonwill triangle is an equilateral triangle with the base b/w the condyles and the apex b/w the central incisors; with 4" side.
- Angle recognized the parabolic arch form.
- Hawley described the arch as a circle. The radius of the circle is the combined width of the 6 anterior teeth; and they are to be placed on this circle. From this circle, an equilateral triangle is made with its base representing the intercondylar distance.
- Angle's Class III malocclusions are least in incidence.
- Most of the cases who visit a doctor for orthodontic treatment are of Angle's Class II nature.

Self Assessment Questions

1. What is curve of spee (COS)?
2. What is normal value of COS?
3. How much space is required to level a deep COS?
4. What is the Andrew's normal molar relationship?
5. What is Flush terminal plane?
6. What is end-on relationship of molars?

Reader's Notes

7

Etiology

◎ **Which are various SYNDROMES causing malocclusion?**

Class II	Class III
• Pierre Robin Synd	• Klienfelter syndrome • CLP osteogenesis imperfecta
• Mouth breathing	• Cleidocranial dysostosis
• Ankylosis of condyles	• Achondroplasia
• Millwaukee brace	• Down's syndrome
• Mandibulofacial dysostosis (Treacher Collin syndrome)	• Bilateral condylar hyperplasia
• Still's disease	• Marfan Synd
• Goldenhar syndrome	• Hyperpituitarism • Craniofacial dystosis (Crouzon's dis.)
• Mobius syndrome	• Gorlin syndrome

◎ **What are the local causes of malocclusion?**

1. Size (microdontia / macrodontia), shape (e.g. peg laterals) and number (partial anodontia / supernumerary teeth, etc.) of teeth.
2. Labial frenum may cause diastema; deflection of path of eruption.
3. Premature loss of primary teeth
4. Prolonged retention of primary teeth.

5. Delayed eruption of permanent teeth
6. Dental caries may lead to space loss.
7. Ankylosis of tooth
8. Improper restorations
9. Abnormal path of eruption

◎ What are the general causes of malocclusion?

1. Heredity
2. Congenital defects = CLP, cleidocranial dysostosis, congenital syphilis, maternal rubella infection, cerebral palsy.
3. Environmental = prenatal / postnatal.
4. Endocrine = hypothyroidism / hypoparathyroidism (delayed eruption of teeth), hypopituitarism (delayed eruption of teeth), hyperthyroidism / hyperparathyroidism (faster tooth eruption).
5. Hyperpituitarism = abnormal growth of jaws especially the mandible.
6. Accidental / trauma
7. Nutritional

◎ What are the Salzmann's causes of malocclusion?

These are congenital; developmental; environmental; functional and genetic causes (CDEFG).

◎ How does the hyperthyroidism affect the orthodontic treatment?

As it can lead to osteoporosis. But in hypothyroidism, there is delayed eruption and abnormal resorption patterns of the teeth.

◎ Which teeth are most commonly missing in the permanent dentition?

U/L 3rd molars; upper lateral incisors; mandibular 2nd premolar; mandibular central incisors; maxillary 2nd premolars in this order of frequency. (Read Butler's field theory.)

◎ Tell some points about labial frenum.

Before the eruption of teeth, it is attached to the alveolar ridge with some fibers attached to the incisive papilla. It moves apically with the eruption of teeth. If it does not move, it may cause midline diastema. It is diagnosed by blanch test. Normally, the frenum has migrated sufficiently superiorly by 10–12 yrs of age.

◎ What are other causes of midline diastema?

These can be mesiodens, tongue thrust or thumb sucking habits, small size of the teeth, e.g. peg laterals, midline cysts, periodontal disease, etc. and UGLY-DUCKLING STAGE.

◎ How will you manage space in the premature loss of deciduous teeth cases?

Space maintenance is not required in maxillary or mandibular anterior region. But, in posterior area, e.g. primary first molar region, the space maintainer is required to avoid loss of space. If second molar is lost before 5–6 yrs of age, the distal shoe appliance is given to guide the eruption of first permanent molar in proper place.

◎ What do you mean by ankylosis?

It is the fusion of root or its part directly to the bone, with the loss of PDL in an area. It can occur due to trauma, intentional replantation of tooth, cleidocranial dysostosis, etc.

◎ How does a submerged tooth develop?

Due to ankylosis of the tooth, the adjoining teeth keep on erupting leading to increase in the alveolar height, while the ankylosed tooth remains at the same level, giving an appearance of submerged tooth.

◎ Explain the term Vogel-Geischt?

When during forceps delivery of a child, trauma occurs to his TMJ area, it may undergo ankylosis. It results in decreased mandibular growth and so a hypoplastic mandible. Here, a severe class II skeletal relation is evident.

◎ **How does the Milwaukee brace affect the growth of mandible?**

It is used for the treatment of scoliosis. It puts continuous pressure on the mandible and retards its growth. A class II relation develops.

◎ **Define habit?**

Habit is defined as the tendency or an act, which has become relatively fixed, a repeated performance and is consistent and easy to perform by the patient.

◎ **What are the different types of habits?**

These can be classified as

1. Useful / harmful
2. Empty / meaningful
3. Pressure / non pressure / biting
4. Compulsive / non-compulsive

◎ **Define the following terms of habits?**

1. Useful / harmful
2. Empty / meaningful
3. Pressure / non pressure / biting
4. Compulsive / non-compulsive

Useful habits = are considered essential for normal function, e.g. proper tongue positioning, swallowing, etc.

Harmful habits = which have a deleterious effect on the dentofacial structures, e.g. tongue thrusting, thumb sucking.

Empty habits = which are not associated with any psychological problems.

Meaningful habits = which has a psychological connection.

Pressure habit = are the sucking habits which apply pressure on the teeth and supporting tissues, e.g. tongue thrusting, thumb sucking.

Non–pressure habits = which do not apply direct forces on the teeth and supporting tissues, e.g. eg mouth breathing.

Biting habits = eg nail biting or lip biting.

Masochistic habits = e.g. which provide tissue damage as incurred by the patient himself, e.g. scraping of gingival tissues, hair pulling.

Compulsive habits = are deep rooted habits which the child does when he feels that his security is in danger or when he feels unsafe.

Non-compulsive habits = which are easily learned and dropped as the child matures.

◎ What are the 3 main factors on which the effect of habit depends for its effect on the dentofacial complex during development?

The 3 factors or the trident of the factors is = frequency, duration and intensity of habit.

◎ Up to what age, the digit sucking may be considered as normal habit?

Up to 3 ½ to 4 yrs age, it can be considered as normal habit.

◎ What is the difference b/w simple tongue thrust and complex tongue thrust?

Teeth come in full ICP during swallowing in simple tongue thrust; but there is gap b/w the teeth in complex TT, in which 7th n ms contract and no temporalis m contraction occurs.

◎ What are the adenoid facies?

It occurs due to chronic mouth breathing habit. The face is long and narrow; blank face; dry lips and gingiva; short and flaccid upper lip and narrow upper arch.

◎ What is lip trap?

When there is increased overjet, the lower lip falls behind the lingual surfaces of upper incisors and on the labial surfaces of lower incisors. With continuous function due to swallowing, etc., the lower lip keeps pressing the incisors in opposite directions and also prevent proper forward growth of the mandible. It contributes in the development of Class II skeleto-dental relation. With the help of the myofunctional appliances, we can treat this condition, e.g. LIP BUMPER, etc.

◎ What is main cause of Class III and Class II malocclusion?

It is hereditary; there is skeletal growth pattern as inherited from either of the parents.

◎ Which conditions have genetic predilection?

These are mainly deep bite, class II div 2 m.o., and class III m.o. Also, cleft lip and / or palate is said to have a genetic basis. CLP is the most common congenital deformation of facial tissues.

◎ How does the class II molar develops in the dentition besides growth problems?

In majority of C2 D1 cases, the maxillary second molar tends to erupt earlier than mandibular second molar (which may be due to space problem in the mandibular arch).

◎ Why do we find maxillary canine blocked out labially in many cases?

Eruption of maxillary first premolar before maxillary canine leads to labial displacement of maxillary canine (and hence crowding) due to lack of space as some of it may get used by maxillary first premolar.

Maxillary 2 are displaced generally LINGUALLY.
Maxillary 3 are displaced generally LABIALLY.
Maxillary 5 are displaced generally PALATALLY.

◎ Which is the most common local cause of malocclusion?

It is the premature fall of primary teeth due to high caries rate.

◎ How do you classify the overbites?

The overbite can be normal bite; closed bite; deep bite; edge–to–edge bite; open bite; traumatic bite.

◎ What are the types of overjet?

Normal; increased; buccal; reverse overjet (i.e. anterior cross bite).

◎ Which all are the types of cross bites?

Anterior cross bite; posterior cross bite; scissor's bite; Brodie's cross bite; telescopic bite; single tooth cross bite; multiple teeth cross bite; buccal / lingual cross bite. It may dental or skeletal in nature.

It can be unilateral or bilateral. In posterior region, it is mostly bilateral cross bite but it gives a presentation of unilateral cross bite when checked in centric occlusion, as the patient tends to close in a convenient intercuspation, due to prematurities.

◎ What do you mean by scissor's bite?

Here, the palatal surface of maxillary tooth is in touch with the buccal surface of the mandibular tooth and vice versa.

◎ What is Brodie's bite?

It is the complete scissor's bite, i.e. mandibular arch is contained in the maxillary arch. It is also known as the telescopic bite.

◎ Which is main cause of Deep bite?

Hereditary

◎ Which is the major etiology of Class II m.o.?

Growth discrepancy.

◎ What is the effect of malocclusion on speech?

Class II div 1 leads to difficult production of bilabial consonants; sibilants are effected in case of anterior open bite cases. Most of these defects are due to DYSLALIC PHENOMENON, i.e. defective articulation due to faulty learning or abnormalities of the external speech organs and not due to lesions of the CNS.

Class III m.o which has an abnormally low tongue position and lethargic tongue function reduces the quality of sibilants.

◎ **How does the forces of masticatory ms differ in horizontal growth pattern to that of vertical growth pattern cases?**

The forces in horizontal growth pattern cases are higher than in the vertical growth cases.

◎ **How does the adenoid facies related to the growth pattern of face in these patients?**

It is dolichofacial, vertical growth pattern. It is due to the continuous open mouth for mouth breathing and so the eruption of the posterior teeth, leading to downward and backward rotation of mandible.

◎ **Is the thumb sucking habit normal in a child?**

It is considered normal up to 3-4 years age. However it should be abolished in the children more than this age. Orthodontic interference for R_x of habits should be started at approx 7-8 years of age.

◎ **Infantile swallowing can be seen normally up to what age?**

Up to 1½ - 2 years.

◎ **What do you understand by the transitional period?**

It is the period of change of infantile swallowing pattern to the adult swallowing pattern during the development of a child. It is said to be completed by the 18 mos. of age of the child.

Self Assessment Questions

1. What is the normal value of over bite?
2. Define over-jet and over bite.
3. Define and classify the open bite.
4. How will you treat a deep bite?
5. What is Telescopic Bite?

Reader's Notes

8

Classification

◎ **Define classification?**

It is defined as a method of grouping together of various conditions having same features into simpler and smaller groups for the ease of description of the condition.

◎ **What are the various incidences of malocclusions according to Angle's classification?**

Angle's Class I = 60%

II = 25%

III = 5%

◎ **Which tooth is the "key to occlusion" according to Angle?**

Maxillary first permanent molar and that too its MB cusp tip.

◎ **What is the normal anatomic landmark to which the MB cusp used in the classifying the malocclusion is related?**

It is the key ridge / the Angle's point. The MB root tip is in line with this point in normal positioned teeth in the maxillary arch. Angle considered this point the most stable point in the arch and considered the relation of the mandibular arch with this position.

◎ **What is Angle's class I molar relation?**

It is the relation of permanent first molars, where the mesiobuccal cusp of maxillary first molar lies in the mesiobuccal groove of mandibular first molar. It is also called normo-occlusion.

◎ **What is Angle's class II molar relation?**

It is the relation of permanent first molars, where the mesiobuccal cusp of maxillary first molar lies mesial to the mesiobuccal groove of mandibular first molar. It is also called disto-occlusion.

◎ **What are the 2 divisions are class II m.o.?**

These are div 1 and div 2. They are further divided in subdivisions.

◎ **What is the difference b/w div 1 and div 2 m.o.**

Div 1 is having the maxillary incisors proclined with increase in overjet. But the div 2 has retroclined incisors with decreased or zero overjet. But the patients have normal perioral ms activity and hence the arch is of squarish shape. But it may have an abnormal backward path of closure. However, both have deep bite.

Div 1 has hyperactive mentalis m and buccinator m; tongue is placed D and B in position. This imbalance leads to contracted upper arch. Upper lip is hypotonic.

◎ **What do you mean by subdivision of malocclusion?**

Subdivision means that class II molar relation is not bilateral but only unilateral. The other side is having class I relation which is the side of subdivision.

◎ **What is Angle's class III molar relation?**

It is the relation of permanent first molars, where the mesiobuccal cusp of maxillary first molar lies distal to the mesiobuccal groove of mandibular first molar. It is also called mesioocclusion.

◎ **What is true class III and the pseudo class III?**

True class III refers to the condition in which there is skeletal mal-relationship. Pseudo / postural class III is the condition in which there is dental / incisal prematurities due to which the mandible has an abnormal forward path of closure for coming in centric occlusion. If this condition is not treated in-time, it may become the true class III in nature with ensuing growth.

◎ What is class IV relation of malocclusion?

It is the additional class included in previous classification. In it, there is Angle's class II relation on one side and the Angle's class III relation on the other side.

◎ Which is the most common type of malocclusion?

Angle's class I is the most common. Skeleto-dental type of condition is the commonest. Lower anterior crowding is the commonest feature.

◎ What are the disadvantages of Angle's classification?

1. It describes the m.o. in AP plane only.
2. It depends on the maxillary first permanent molar. If this tooth is missing, the classification is not possible.
3. It describes the condition only according to the dental parameters. It has no provision of a skeletal classification.
4. It cannot find the cause of the condition.
5. It cannot be applied to the primary dentition.

◎ What is the skeletal classification of malocclusion?

1. Skeletal class I = there is normal AP relation of maxillary and mandibular bases. The ANB angle is 0–4 degrees.
2. Skeletal class II = there is either maxillary prognathism or mandibular retrognathism, or a combination of both in the AP dimension. The ANB angle is more than 5 degrees.
3. Skeletal class III = there is either maxillary retrognathism or maxillary retrognathism, or a combination of both in the AP dimension. The ANB angle is less than zero degrees.

PS: the malrelation can also be classified as dental; skeletal and dento-skeletal. However, the malocclusion is always a combination of both and so most of the time it is dento-skeletal.

◎ What are the Lischer's modification of the Angle's classification?

It has given the synonyms to the different classes of Angle's classification. The class I, II, III are known as normocclusion, distocclusion and mesiocclusion respectively.

◎ **What is the incisor classification?**

It was described by British Society of Orthodontics.

1. Type I = the incisal edges of lower incisors are just below the cinguli of the upper incisors, without touching them.
2. Type II = the incisal edges of lower incisors are posterior to the cinguli of the upper incisors.
3. Type III = the incisal edges of lower incisors are anterior to the cinguli of the upper incisors.

◎ **Which is most common problem found in the malocclusion?**

It is mostly crowding of teeth, especially of lower incisors. Imbrication is the other term given to lower incisors crowding. It is the main basis of Peck and Peck ratio, which helps to find out the discrepancy in MD width and facio-lingual dimension thickness of these teeth.

◎ **What is the normal molar relation according to Andrew's laws?**

It has three features.

Here the mesiobuccal cusp of maxillary first molar lies in the mesiobuccal groove of mandibular first molar. Also the mesiolingual cusp of maxillary first molar lies in the central fossa of mandibular first molar. Distal marginal ridge of maxillary first molar occludes with the mesial marginal ridge of mandibular second molars.

◎ **What is the normal relation of the mesiobuccal root of maxillary first molar according to Angle?**

MB root lies in relation to the **key ridge,** i.e. the lowermost point of the zygoma bone.

◎ **What is Simon's Law of Canines?**

Orbital plane (i.e. perpendicular to FHP under the pupil) passes through distal third of upper canines.

In **class I canine relation**, mesial incisal ridge of maxillary canine overlaps the distal incisal ridge of mandibular canine. Also, the tip of upper canine falls in the embrasure between lower canine and first premolar.

In class II canine relation, the mesial cusp ridge of upper canine lies mesial to the embrasure b/w lower canine and first premolar.

In class III canine relation, the mesial cusp ridge of upper canine lies distal to the embrasure b/w lower canine and first premolar.

◎ What is Simon's classification?

Here, 3 planes are used for classifying the condition which are: FHP, orbital plane and midsagittal plane.

Dimension	Plane	If towards plane	If away from plane
Vertical	FHP	Attraction	Abstraction
AP	Orbital	Protraction	Retraction
Transverse	midsagittal	Contraction	Distraction

◎ What is Dewey's modification of Angle's class I malocclusion classification?

Type 1 Crowding

Type 2 Spacing

Type 3 Anterior Cross Bite

Type 4 Posterior Cross Bite

Type 5 Disturbed Molar Relation Due To Early Loss Of Primary Second Molars.

◎ What are the Dewey's modification of Angle's class III m.o?

Type 1 Upper and lower incisors are edge to edge

Type 2 Lower incisors are lingual to the upper incisors, i.e. normal relation

Type 3 Lower incisors are labial to the upper incisors, i.e. cross bite

◎ What are various relations of incisors in class II div 2 m.o?

Type 1 Only upper centrals are lingually inclined and laterals are labially inclined

Type 2 Upper centrals and laterals are lingually inclined while canines are labially inclined

Type 3 Upper centrals, laterals and canines are lingually inclined

◎ What is Bennett's classification?

According to this classification:

1. Class I is due to local causes
2. Class II is due to developmental defects in either arch.
3. Class III is due to abnormal relation of both arches, etc.

◎ What do you mean by the terms transversion and torsiversion?

Transversion is the transposition of two teeth, i.e. exchange in the position during eruption. Torsiversion of teeth is the rotation of a tooth around its long axis.

◎ What are the features to be studied according to Ackermann-Proffit (A–P) classification?

1. Alignment / symmetry = normal / crowding / spacing
2. Profile = straight / convex / concave / anterior divergent / posterior divergent.
3. Type (in transverse dimension) = midline; buccal / palatal posterior cross bite; skeletal / dental; unilateral / bilateral.
4. Class (sagittal dimension) = Angle's class I, II, III; anterior cross bite; skeletal / dental; overjet.
5. Bite (vertical dimension) = over bite; deep bite; open bite; skeletal/ dental; growth; face height.

◎ How many groups are there in A–P classification?

Nine groups.

◎ What are the advantages of A–P classification over Angle's classification?

It describes the condition in all the 3-dimensions; describes skeletal or dental conditions; growth pattern; and the cause of the condition.

◎ What is Cephalic Index?

It is = Breadth of the cranium × 100 / length of cranium.

1. Dolichocephalic: 75 or less
2. Mesocephalic : 75-80
3. Brachycephalic: 80 or more

Self Assessment Questions

1. What are various individual-tooth malpositions?
2. What is facial index?
3. What are various growth patterns?
4. Define the term INDEX.
5. What is the Treatment Priority Index (TPI)?
6. What is the Index of orthodontic treatment needs (IOTN)?

◎ What is the Pseudo class III malocclusion?

Class III molar relation is seen due to the deviated path (anteriorly) of closure due to occlusal prematurities; it is Skeletal class I, but may change to true class III if not treated in time due to unhindered growth of mandible. So the prematurity, eg cross bite should be treated as soon as possible or by grinding of the teeth.

◎ What is a True class III relation?

It is a skeletal class III relation due to abnormal growth pattern. It may due to maxillary retrognathism / hypoplasia or mandibular prognathism or a combination of both. It should be treated as soon as possible. The maxillary retrognathism is treated with Delaire's face mask; the mandibular prognathism is treated with chin cup.

Chin cup helps to redirect / interfere the growth of overgrowing mandible.

However, due to long term growth, the retention period is very long till the completion of growth phase, i.e. approx 18 yrs of age.

Surgical intervention to treat these conditions should be done only after the cessation of growth, i.e. 18 yrs of age, to minimize the chances of relapse.

◎ **What are the clinical feature of Class II Div. 2 m.o?**

Maxillary Central incisors lingually inclined and the lateral incisors are labially inclined. Backward path of closure; Horizontal growth patterns; Increased freeway space and so Closed / deep bite. Muscular pattern of lips and cheeks is normal.

◎ **Why there is a deep bite in class II div 1 and div 2?**

It is due to the unobstructed eruption of lower incisors, as the incisal edges are placed distally to the cinguli of upper incisors.

◎ **What is the difference in the path of closure b/w class II div 2 m.o. and pseudo–class III m.o.?**

It is backward in the former, and forward in the later as guided by upper incisors position.

◎ **What is Sunday bite?**

Bite achieved by patient by deliberately bringing his mandible forward in Class II Div. 1 to improve his esthetics.

◎ **Which facial ms are hyperactive in Class II div 2 m.o.?**

Upper lip is hyperactive in this condition, but not always.

◎ **What do you mean by bimaxillary protrusion and bimaxillary prognathism?**

Bimaxillary protrusion means that the teeth are proclined, while their bases normally related to each other and the cranial base. But, bimaxillary prognathism means that the skeletal bases are placed forward with respect to cranial base, their mutual relationship may be quite normal. (SNA, SNB may be increased; ANB is normal.)

◎ **What is the difference b/w the skeletal and dental malocclusion conditions?**

Skeletal m.o is the disharmony b/w the jaws bases in all the 3–D of the space. Eg prognathism or retrognathism of the jaws. But, the dental m.o means that the jaw bases are normally related, while only dental positions are at fault, e.g. crowding, rotations, cross bites, etc.

However, most of the malocclusions are a combination of both, i.e. are mostly skeleto-dental type.

◎ Which facial ms are at fault in C2, D1 m.o.?

It is hypotonic (U) lip, and hyperactive mentalis m.

Malocclusion	Abnormal ms activity
Class I; class II div 2	Normal ms
Class II div 1; class III	Tongue is in floor of the mouth; so V–shaped arch
Class II div 1	Lower lip is more active; lip trap; hyperactive mentalis ms; upper lip is hypotonic
Class III	Upper lip is more active
Class II div 2	Exaggerated curve of spee; tooth guidance / deviated path of closure by incisors
Pseudo class III	Anterior path of closure due to premature contacts.

◎ How does the ms activity differ in the normal and abnormal swallowing patterns?

Normal swallowing	Abnormal swallowing
Only lateral and medial pterygoids; middle temporalis and anterior and posterior masseter fibers show moderate activity.	Heavy mentalis and lip (labii superioris and inferioris ms) activity; dominant posterior temporalis and masseter fibers activity; increased hyoid ms action

◎ Why there is narrow upper arch in class II div 1 m.o.?

In this m.o., there is low lying position of tongue and so its effect on the lingual side of the teeth is decreased, while the buccinator ms on buccal side has a normal or increased contraction leading to contraction or narrow upper arch.

◎ What is Simon's law of canine?

It is used to describe the normal position of the maxillary canine in the arch. According to this law, a perpendicular drawn on FHP from the inferior most point of the orbital margin should pass through the distal 3rd of maxillary canines in class I cases. But if this perpendicular passes distal to the canine, it is class II. If it is mesial to the canine, it is class III.

◎ Why there is deep bite in class II div 1 and div 2 m.o.?

It is due to the overeruption of incisors as there is no prevention due to increased or decreased overjet. In normal cases, the incisal edges of lower incisors are just below the cinguli of upper incisors.

◎ What is the normal / ideal relation of upper and lower canines?

The cusp tip of upper canine should fall in line of the buccal embrasure of lower canine and premolar.

◎ What is the position of tongue in class II div 1 m.o.?

It is placed downward and backward in the oral cavity, as compared to the normal tongue with its tip resting at rugae area and on the edges of lower incisors.

◎ What are the muscle's problems as seen generally in class II div 1 m.o.?

There is hyperactive mentalis m, lower lip trap and hypoactive upper lip. The lips are incompetent. It may be due to increased overjet also.

◎ If in a patient, upper and lower first permanent molars are missing, how do you classify the malocclusion?

It is done with the help of permanent canines. The mesial incisal edge of upper canine overlaps the distal incisal edge of lower canines in class I relations. If the incisal tip of upper canine is mesial to the embrasure of lower 3, 4 teeth, it is ka class II relation. If it is distal to the embrasure, it is ka class III relation.

◎ What is the significance of key-ridge.

The mesiobuccal root of maxillary first permanent molar is in line with this ridge in its normal position in the maxillary arch as described by Angle. Key ridge is the inferior most point of the anterior border of the zygoma as seen in the lateral cephalogram. If MB root of the maxillary first permanent molar is mesial to the key ridge, it leads to the class II position.

◎ What do you mean by Jackson's triad?

It describes the goals of the orthodontic treatment, i.e. esthetics, stability and health of investing tissues, along with the functional harmony of the anatomic structures.

Self Assessment Questions

1. What are different types of incisors relationship in Angle's Class II Div 2 cases?
2. Simon's classification of malocclusion in 3-dimensions, i.e.

   Abstraction/Attraction

   Protraction/Retraction

   Contraction/Distraction
3. What are the goals of orthodontic R_x?
4. What is orbital law of canine?
5. What is Angle's class IV relationship of molars?

Reader's Notes

9

Diagnosis

◎ **What are the essential diagnostic aids?**

Various essential diagnostic aids are: case history; clinical examination; study models; photos; and x–rays, i.e. IOPA, bitewing and OPG.

◎ **What are supplemental diagnostic aids?**

These are: specialized r/g, i.e. lateral cephalograms and occlusal; EMG; hand–wrist R/G; BMR; endocrine status; occlusograms and Kesling's diagnostic set-up.

◎ **What do you mean by wax bite record or wafer bite or the squash bite?**

The patient is asked to bite on the 1–2 layers of the soft base plate wax in the centric occlusion without perforating it. This helps to reorient the upper and lower casts properly in the articulator or the records.

◎ **What do you mean by the term milestones?**

Certain developmental features appear at certain time period of age as the child grows, e.g. rolling, crawling, standing, walking, teething, speaking, etc.

These are ka the milestones. The importance of knowledge of mile stones is that any delay in development gives an indication of slow growth of the patient.

◎ What do you mean by delayed eruption?

If a tooth fails to erupt more than 6 months beyond its scheduled time, it is said to be a delayed eruption.

◎ What do you mean by ectopic eruption?

If a tooth erupts at other position rather than its scheduled position, it is known as ectopic eruption.

◎ What is the importance of recording name, age, address, SE status and religion of the patient?

By these information, we can contact the patient if required; can know the growth status of the patient especially females, which can be helpful to us during the treatment; by SE status, we can know the cooperation and eating habits of the patient.

◎ Why medical history is important for every patient?

It helps us to plan the treatment for the patient keeping in mind his systemic conditions.

1. If diabetes = it should be controlled, because healing is difficult and poor in these patients. Also infections can occur.
2. If blood dyscrasias = problems can be encountered during extractions and scaling, etc.
3. If endocrine problems = e.g. hyperthyroidism, orthodontic treatment is contraindicated.
4. If TB, HIV, Hep B infections = special precautions are required.
5. If rheumatic fever = antibiotic coverage is indicated.

◎ How do you classify the physique of the patient?

Physique has been divided as

1. Ectomorphic = tall, lean and thin
2. Endomorphic = broad and short
3. Mesomorphic = average; in b/w the above two.

◎ Which are the various forms of head and face?

Various forms of head are–dolichocephalic (long and narrow); brachycephalic (short and broad); mesocephalic (in b/w the above two).

It also gives an indication of width and form of dental arches of the patient.

Face has been classified as – leptoprosopic (long and narrow); euryprosopic (short and broad); and mesoprosopic (in b/w the above two).

◎ What is the cephalic index?

It is the ratio of transverse diameter of skull to the AP length of skull in %age. The normal value is 75–80 %, i.e. mesocephalic; < 75 % means dolichocephalic and > 80 % means brachycephalic.

◎ What is a profile? What are the different types of profile?

Profile is the outline of the face when seen from the lateral side of the patient. Different profiles are straight, convex and concave. Also, it may be anteriorly divergent and posteriorly divergent.

Profile is observed by joining the points N, A, and Pog which tells about the straight, convex and concave nature. Convex profile is seen in class II cases and the concave profile is seen in Class III cases.

If a line joining the points N and Pog inclines anteriorly, it is anteriorly-divergent. But if it inclines posteriorly, it is posterior-divergent. The patient is placed with his FHP parallel to floor while checking the profile.

◎ What are the different relations of lips to be observed during clinical examination?

Lips may be competent, incompetent, potentially incompetent (i.e. the normal lips which cannot form lip seal due to protruded incisors) and everted (i.e. hypertrophied lips due to weak ms tonicity). At rest, there is a normal gap of 2 mm b/w upper and the lower teeth. Redundant lips are seen in patient having very small FMA angle. Skeletal deep bite/horizontal growth pattern.

◎ How do you assess the method of respiration whether oral or nasal?

It can be judged by: mirror test, cotton test, water test, etc.

◎ What are the paths of closure in class II div 2, pseudo class III and in cases of narrow maxillary arch with premature contacts?

Backward path of closure in Class II div 2; forward path of closure in pseudo class III and lateral path of closure in narrow maxillary arch.

◎ What is the main advantage of study models during the clinical examination of the patient?

The occlusal relationship can be studied from lingual side also.

◎ What is the role of bite wing r/g?

It helps us to detect the proximal caries, any secondary caries and the gingival margins of the fillings.

◎ What is the advantage of OPG during the diagnosis?

OPG shows the mandible, maxilla and all the teeth in one view. It gives us complete information about the periapical areas of the teeth, internal morphology of the bones, any pathology like cysts etc. in the bones. The main advantage lies in that it requires less radiation dose as compared to the full mouth IOPA series. It is easy to store also.

◎ What is the use of hand–wrist r/g during the diagnosis?

By studying development status of various bones in this area, we are able to judge the growth status of the patient. Eg skeletal maturity index is based on the study of the bones of hand. Three most common bones to be studied are – hamate hook, pisiform and sesamoid.

◎ In which condition, the orthodontic treatment is contraindicated?

In Marfan's syndrome and hyperthyroidism.

◎ What is Kesling's diagnostic setup?

The teeth of the patient's cast are cut and rearranged in wax to find out TSALD and the most suitable treatment options eg extraction, stripping, etc. (TSALD = Tooth-Size, Arch-Length, Discrepancy).

◎ What are a few features of Soft tissue examinations?

1. VERTICALLY, face can be divided in 3 parts in 1: 1 ratio as
   a. Upper third = from hair line to root of the nose/ glabella
   b. Middle third = from root of the nose/glabella to subnasal
   c. Lower third = from subnasal to lowermost point on chin.
2. Transversely, face can be divided in 5 equal parts.
3. **Width of the nose** is equal to medial intercanthal distance.
4. **Width of the mouth** = distance b/w medial limbus of one eye to other.
5. Subnasal to vermillion border of lower lip = vermillion border of lower lip to lowermost point on chin.
6. Ratio of the distance of 'Subnasal to the junction of upper and lower lips" to the distance from the junction of upper and lower lips to lowermost point on chin = 1:2

◎ What are the various lip relations?

1. Competent, i.e. upper and lower lips are in touch or with a maximum gap of 2 mm at rest.
2. Incompetent, i.e. both the lips are not in touch with each other at rest. It is mostly due to short upper lip.
3. Potentially incompetent = the lips length is normal but the upper lip is not in touch with lower lip due to protrusive incisors. This condition gets corrected when the upper incisors are retracted during the treatment.

◎ What are the various uses of the study casts?

It helps to give us the following information:

1. Classification of m.o.
2. Overjet and overbite

3. Upper to lower midline relationship.
4. Palatal contour: sagittal and transverse.
5. Teeth clinically present
6. Tooth measurements
7. Arch form and symmetry
8. Incisor midline to the jaw midline.
9. Horizontal and Vertical tooth malpositions
10. Abnormal tooth morphology
11. Arch length determinations
12. Axial inclination of teeth
13. Facets of wear
14. Muscle attachments
15. Diagnostic set up if needed
16. Functional analysis
17. Lingual occlusal analysis.

◎ What is the specification for the cephalostat to take a lateral cephalogram?

It is 75-80 kvp; 7-8 mA; 0.8 sec; at a distance of 5 feet from the midsagittal plane.

◎ What is the advantage of cephalography?

It is used to study on the following:

1. Growth and development
2. Craniofacial abnormalities
3. Facial types and skeletal patterns
4. Case analysis, diagnosis and treatment planning
5. Progress of the case and treatment.
6. Functional analysis

Self Assessment Questions

1. Define the terms, diagnosis, prognosis and treatment plan.
2. How do you calculate cephalic index?

3. How will you calculate the facial index?
4. Which are the 5 parts in which face can be divided transversely?
5. What is nasolabial angle?
6. What are the different parts of an ideal study model?
7. What are different specifications of base formation of a study model?
8. Why FHP is called so?
9. What do you mean by dental and skeletal open bite?
10. What are the causes of anterior open bite?

Reader's Notes

10

Cast Analysis

◎ **What is an impression?**

It is the negative replica of the oral tissues.

◎ **What do you mean by cast / model?**

It is the positive replica of the oral tissues. It is made by pouring a suitable material in the impression.

◎ **What is a study model?**

It is the essential diagnostic aid used in orthodontics. It helps in the viewing the occlusion from all the aspects especially the lingual.

◎ **What are the parts of a study model?**

It has 2 main parts, i.e. anatomic and the artistic. The ratio of anatomic to the artistic part is 3:1.

◎ **What is Simon's gnathostatic model?**

In it, the base of upper model is parallel to the FHP. It is difficult to make. It gives us the readily visualization of angulation of teeth to the FHP. It was designed in 1926.

◎ **What are the advantages of a cast?**

There is no requirement of the patient for lab work; occlusion can be seen from the lingual; act as pretreatment record; used for comparison of the results, etc.

◎ What are the types of casts?

Casts can be working cast; study cast; refractory cast; diagnostic casts.

Working cast = is the cast on which simple lab work, eg wax up, orthodontic appliances fabrication, etc. can be done.

Study cast = which is used for keeping as records and for preliminary study of the condition and for discussion with the patient and other colleagues.

Refractory cast = it is prepared in special material which can withstand high temperatures. It is used in labs to form castings for FPD, etc. at high temperatures.

Diagnostic casts = are used for surveying purpose and for other diagnosis reasons.

◎ What is Ashley Howe's analysis?

It helps to determine whether there is need of tooth removal or not during orthodontic treatment.

If PMBAW

≤ 37%	Extraction
37-44%	Border Line
> 44%	Non-Extraction

◎ What is Bolton's Analysis?

It uses the mesiodistal dimensions of various teeth and the relation of upper and lower teeth to determine the requirement of extraction or interdental stripping for alignment of teeth.

Anterior Ratio = 77.2%

Overall Ratio = 91.3%

◎ How the Peck and Peck Ratio is used during diagnosis?

Here, the ratio of MD width and the BL dimension is calculated to determine the discrepancy in size. **Only lower incisors** are used in this analysis because **crowding** is most common in this region.

(L) C.I. = 88-92%

(L) L.I. = 90-95%

◎ **According to Proffit's space analysis, how do you decide whether to extract or not in treating a case?**

If TSALD is	0-5 mm	=	non-extraction case
	5-9 mm	=	Borderline case
	> 9 mm	=	Extraction case

◎ **What is Carey's analysis?**

If crowding is	0-2.5 mm	=	non extraction case
	2.5-4 mm	=	second premolar extraction case
if more than	4 mm	=	first premolar extraction case

However, it is an obsolete analysis nowadays.

◎ **Which analyses help us to determine the arch width or the requirement of expansion?**

Pont's index; Ashley–Howe's index; Linder–Harth index.

◎ **Which analyses help us to determine the arch length discrepancy?**

Profitt's analysis; Nance–Carey's analysis; Total space analysis; Tweed's analysis.

◎ **Which analyses help us to determine the MD dimensions of 3, 4, 5 teeth?**

Tanaka–Johnston's analysis; Moyer's mixed dentition analysis;

◎ **Which analyses use radiographs for calculations?**

Tweed's analysis uses lateral cephalogram; Nance's analysis and Huckaba's analysis use IOPA x-rays.

◎ **Which analysis uses a probability table for calculating the total MD dimension of 3, 4, 5 teeth?**

Moyer's analysis uses a table at 75 % probability level.

◎ **Which analyses help us to determine the amount of stripping required during the treatment for alignment?**

Peck and Peck ratio; Bolton's analysis.

◎ **Which analyses help us to determine the palatal depth?**

Korkhaus analysis.

Self Assessment Questions

1. What is PONT's index?
2. What is LINE of occlusion according to Angle?
3. What is Huckaba's analysis?
4. Describe Tanaka-Johnston's analysis?
5. Describe PONT's analysis?

Reader's Notes

11

Cephalometrics

◎ **Which are the main reference planes used in the cephalometrics?**

- Main reference plane used in Downs analysis = FHP
- Reference plane used in Steiners analysis = SN plane
- Reference plane used in Ricketts analysis is = Anatomic FHP

◎ **Why the SN plane is mostly used in the growth and development research studies?**

It is considered as the most stable plane; it is defined by the true skeletal landmarks. It is easiest to establish; with minimum error. Its growth is earliest to be completed.

◎ **What is the importance of postural resting position?**

It is the most stable dental relationship throughout life and is least affected by growth disturbances and the environmental influences.

What is the extension of FHP?

◎ FHP extends from = Po–Or

◎ **What is the Bjork's sum and what is its significance?**

Bjork's sum = N S Ar + S Ar Go + Ar Go Me = 396° ± 6°

If Bjork's Sum < 390° = Horizontal growth pattern

If Bjork's Sum > 400° = Vertical growth pattern

◎ **What is Jarabak's ratio and what does it signify?**

Jarabak ratio = PFH/AFH % = 62-65%

If Jarabak ratio > 65% = Horizontal growth pattern

If Jatrabak ratio < 62 % = Vertical growth pattern

◎ **What are the few important technical norms of cephalometry?**

- Acceptable magnification on a cephalogram is 5-7%.
- It technical specification of the machine are at 80 KV / 8mA / 0.8 sec.
- Distance of film from midsagittal plane in ceph = 18 cm
- Distance of X-ray source to midsagittal plane = 5 Feet
- Mainly cephalogram taken is of left side of head.

◎ **What is the normal ratio of cephalometric upper and lower anterior facial heights?**

Ratio of UAFH to LAFH = 45 : 55, i.e. 1.2. The UAFH is N-ANS and LAFH is ANS-Me.

◎ **How can you say that the cephalogram is a standardized radiograph?**

It is because each R/G is taken with the patient positioned at the constant distance, and the exposure factors are kept the same. So it is a reproducible and standardized method.

◎ **What is the constant distance and other parameters in this technique?**

Distance b/w x-ray source and midsagittal plane is 5 feet; taken at 80 kvp; 8 mA and 0.8 sec exposure time.

◎ **What are the anatomic and the derived landmarks?**

Anatomic landmarks are the actual anatomic structures of the skull. Derived landmarks are obtained secondarily from anatomic structures.

◎ Define nasion, orbitale, sella, points A and B; pogion, menton points.

Nasion = most anterior point on the frontonasal suture.

Orbitale = lower most point on the inferior bony margin of the orbit.

Porion = is the superior most point on the upper margin of external auditory meatus.

Sella = it is the mid point of the sella turcica.

Point A = point A is the deepest point in the midline b/w ANS and alveolar crest.

Point B = is deepest point in the midline b/w alveolar crest and mental process.

Pogonion = most anterior point of the bony chin in the midline.

Menton = lower most point on the symphysis or bony chin.

◎ What is Tweed's triangle?

It is a diagnostic triangle in cephalogram having FMA, FMIA, and IMPA angles. The normal values of these angles are 25, 65 and 90 degrees. FMA gives an idea of growth pattern. FMIA indicates the esthetic value.

◎ Which are various soft tissue lines used in cephalometrics?

These are = (MRSH)

1. **Merrifield's** line = line passing from soft tissue pognion to the most prominent lip, whether upper or lower.
2. **Rickett's** line = line passing from soft tissue pognion to the tip of the nose.
3. **Steiner's** line = line passing from soft tissue pognion to the centre of the S-shaped curve formed by passing from nose to the upper lip.
4. **Holdaway's** line = line passing from soft tissue pognion to the most prominent point on upper lip.

◎ Which horizontal planes are most commonly used in cephalometry?

These from top to bottom are: SN, FHP, PP, OP and MP. According to Sassouni, all these planes meet at the base of occipital bone just behind the foramen magnum in a well - proportioned face. In a vertically growing face, they meet in front of F. magnum; while in horizontally growing faces, they tend to meet far behind the cranium or do not meet at all.

◎ What do the SNA and SNB angles signify?

SNA tells us the AP relation of maxilla to the cranial base. SNB tells us the same relation b/w mandible and the cranial base. Normal values of SNA and SNB are 82° and 80° respectively.

- An increased SNA denotes maxillary prognathism
- An decreased SNA denotes maxillary retrognathism
- An increased SNB denotes mandibular prognathism.
- A decreased SNB denotes mandibular retrognathism.

◎ What is the significance of ANB angle in orthodontics?

ANB angle describes the anteroposterior relationship of the maxillary and mandibular bases to each other. Its normal value is 0–4 degrees.

If more than 5, it shows a skeletal class II pattern; and if it is less than zero degrees, it shows a skeletal class III pattern.

However, it does not describe which skeletal base is the cause of this skeletal discrepancy. It can only be judged by correlating the angles SNA and SNB.

◎ What is cervical vertebra maturation index?

Status of growth of a patient can be evaluated by assessing the status of development of cervical vertebrae from the cephalogram. Various stages are given in the following table.

Stage	Growth Remaining	Shape	Inferior border
Initiation	80–100 %	Wedge	Flat
Acceleration	65–85 %	Rectangular	Slight concavity
Transition	25–65 %	Rectangular	Slight concave
Deceleration	10–25%	Square	Distinct concave
Maturation	5–10 %	Square	Accentuated concavity
Completion	0–little	Vertical Dim > hori.	Deep concavities

◎ **How does the Hand wrist R/G help in assessing the growth status of the patient?**

Here, the growth and development of hamate, pisiform and sesamoid bones is evaluated.

1. Absence of **sesamoid bone** at average onset of puberty in a female => retardation of pubertal development.
2. Initiation ossification of **pisiform and hook of hamate** = preceded peak growth in most males and females.
3. Initial ossification of sesamoid of thumb and advanced ossification of HH coincided with peak growth in most M and that was true in only about half of the F.

◎ **Which are the 8 carpel bones in the human wrist?**

These are scaphoid; lunate; triquetral; pisiform; trapezium, trapezoid, capitate and hamate.

◎ **How does the growth status of a patient affect the treatment plan?**

Treatment given during growing age is more rapid and stable. Also, certain modalities, eg myofunctional therapy is possible during growth spurts stage, taking full advantage of growth; the effects are more skeletal; rapid and stable. Similarly expansion, serial extraction, orthopedic therapy with delaire face mask and chin cups is better during growth spurts. Females should be treated 2–3 yrs before the males, since the growth spurts are advanced in females.

◎ **What are the different methods of gaining space?**

1. **Expansion** = 1 mm / mm of expansion can be gained in intercanine region.
2. **Reproximation** = 0.5 mm per interdental area, i.e. 0.25 mm per tooth surface.
3. **Distalization of molars** = up to 5-6 mm space can be gained on each side of the upper arch. It is not possible in lower arch, where only distal tipping is achieved due to dense bone.
4. **Protrusion of incisors** = 1 mm / mm of protrusion can be gained, i.e. 0.5 mm / side of the arch.
5. **Derotation** of molars / PMs = rotated posteriors occupy more space.
6. **Uprighting of incisors** = MD inclined anteriors occupy more space.
7. **Uprighting of molars**
8. **Extraction** = 7 mm / side of space can be gained by removal of first premolars.

◎ **What is stripping / reproximation?**

It is the removal of enamel from the mesial and distal surfaces of a tooth. It is done if the MD dimension of the teeth are not proportionate to labio-lingual dimension as indicated by Peck and Peck ratio, or by Bolton's ratio. **Stripping** is indicated if TSALD = 0–2.5 mm.

- Not > 50% enamel thickness should be reduced, i.e. 0.25 mm / surface.
- Immediate **Fluoride** application is recommended to replenish the surface layer of enamel with Fluoride.
- ARS, i.e. **air rotor stripping** is better than the hand strips.

Self Assessment Questions

1. What is the nasolabial angle?
2. What do you mean by Gonial angle and FMA?
3. Who discovered the cephalostat?
4. What are various skeletal and dental parameters evaluated in DOWN's analysis and Steiner's analysis?
5. Which parameters angles help us to determine the growth pattern of the face?
6. What do you mean by serial cephalography?
7. Why FHP has been given this name?

Reader's Notes

12

Preventive Orthodontics

◎ **What are the various procedures undertaken in preventive orthodontics?**

1. Parent education.
2. Caries control and oral hygiene
3. Care of the primary dentition
4. Oral habits
5. Space maintenance
6. Eruption of the permanent teeth
7. Occlusal equilibration of prematurities
8. Removal of supernumerary teeth
9. Treatment of abnormal frenal attachments.

- Caries can lead to loss of arch length by mesial migration if the caries is on the proximal surfaces, so the teeth should be filled as soon as possible.
- Primary teeth are the best space maintainers, so they should be preserved until the permanent teeth erupt in the oral cavity.
- No space maintainer is required in the maxillary anterior segment, since the normal growth and development leads to an increase in intercanine width.
- Caries can be controlled by improving oral hygiene, by topical application of fluorides, by using fluoridated tooth pastes, and by pit and fissure sealants.

- Supernumerary teeth eg mesiodens, should be extracted as soon as possible, as they block the space of the permanent teeth, deflect the path of the erupting teeth to abnormal positions.
- Occlusal prematurities should be removed to avoid development of any deviations in the path of closure of the mandible. It can lead to the development of abnormal habits eg bruxism.
- The shedding of the primary teeth should be symmetric on the both sides of the jaws. It helps to avoid the development of midline shift. The cause should be identified and eliminated.
- Abnormal soft tissue and frenal attachments should be eliminated, as they cause deflected path of eruption of the teeth. Ankyloglossia leads to problems in speech and swallowing.
- Space maintenance should be done to prevent any arch length loss and to maintain the space for the eruption of the permanent teeth.
- Special nipples should be advised to the infants for drinking the milk so that the sucking force does not fall on the developing and erupting teeth and the maxillary anterior alveolar process.

Self Assessment Questions

1. What is the R_x of abnormal frenum attachment?
2. How do you diagnose a low attached maxillary frenum?
3. What is the R_x of ankyloglossia?
4. Which space maintainer is required if mandibular primary second molar is lost at 5 years of age?
5. Which is the best space maintainer?
6. What is Roche's appliance?
7. What are various methods of caries prevention and control?

Reader's Notes

13

Interceptive Orthodontics

◎ **What is serial extraction?**

It is defined as the planned removal of certain primary and permanent teeth. It is also ka guidance of occlusion now.

◎ **What are the ideal cases for serial extraction?**

a) 8½ - 9½ year age (Growing period)

b) TSALD$\geq$ 10 mm

c) Skeletal Class I relations.

◎ **What is the main side effect of serial extraction?**

It causes lingual tipping of mandibular incisors and so the deep bite development. It causes loss of arch length from the anterior.

◎ **How does the loss of arch length occur in serial extraction cases?**

It occurs both from anterior and posterior. It occurs by lingual tipping of the incisors under lip pressure after extraction of canines, and by mesial movement of the posterior teeth and forces of closure of mandible.

◎ **Which are the teeth extracted during serial extraction?**

The main teeth removed are C, D, 4 from each quadrant. These teeth are removed after a gap of ***6–12 months*** depending on the status of eruption of teeth.

◎ How does the intercanine width is affected in serial extraction?

This process is started during 8–9 yrs of age; and after a gap of 6–12 months, the teeth are removed in succession. It is during this time, the intercanine, (I/C) width changes. In mandibular arch, the I/C width changes at approx 9 yrs age so it is not affected by removal of mandibular primary canine.

But in maxillary arch, the I/C width increases in 11–12 yrs age, so if maxillary canine is removed before the increase of I/C width, then the maxillary arch remains narrow. So in especially maxillary arch, the serial extraction should be done carefully.

◎ What are the different sequences of serial extraction?

Nance's; and Tweed's processes follow C,D,4 sequence, but Dewel's process follows D,4,C sequence. However, teeth should be extracted according to clinical and radiographic progress and findings.

◎ Can we achieve the proper alignment with Serial Extraction?

We cannot achieve proper alignment with it, so in most of the cases, generally full fixed orthodontic treatment is always required. But it decreases the severity of developing condition/malpositions.

◎ What is the advantage of Serial Extraction?

It helps in natural shifting of teeth during the eruption of teeth in almost normal positions and so stability of the treatment is increased.

◎ How much space is needed for the leveling of curve of Spee?

A space of 1 mm / mm of the depth of Curve of Spee is required.

◎ How much space is needed for the uprighting of lower incisors?

It is 0.4 mm / degree / side, i.e. 0.8 mm / degree of the uprighting.

◎ How much space do you get by maxillary expansion?

In canine region, we get 1 mm / mm of expansion; in premolar region, we get 0.5 mm / mm and; in molar region, we get only 0.25 mm / mm of space. On an average, we gain 1.57 mm/mm of arch perimeter with the expansion.

◎ What is the functional cross bite?

Here, the mandible while coming in the C.O. position, is deflected anteriorly due to premature contacts in the incisor region leading to Class III condition. If checked in the rest position, the skeletal relationship of both jaws is Class I. It should be treated as soon as possible, as it can lead to true Class III relationship if left unattended due to growth of mandible.

◎ Interception of habits is important for proper development of dentofacial relation. Comment.

Habits disturb the balance of the muscular forces responsible for the proper development of the dentofacial relations. Eg mouth breathing lowers the mandible and tongue and can lead to narrow arches and long face patterns.

◎ What is the effect of hypertrophic adenoids and tonsils on the dental occlusion?

With this condition, the patient resorts to mouth breathing. It causes rotation of mandible in a D and B direction and so a gap is created b/w the occlusal surfaces of U and L teeth, in which the posterior teeth are free to erupt. It increases the facial height. Also, the tongue occupies the lower position in the mouth, thus balance of the muscles is lost. It leads to constricted upper arch and so development of posterior cross bite and the protrusion of maxillary incisors.

◎ When should be a cross bite needs correction?

It should be treated as soon as possible, as it is an obstruction to the proper growth of the jaws. A case of pseudo- class III should be corrected as it may lead to true class III if it is not treated, due to ensuing uninterrupted growth of mandible.

Self Assessment Questions

1. What do you mean by space regaining?
2. What are various space regainers?
3. What other procedures are indicated in interceptive orthodontics?
4. How do you treat a case of mouth breathing?
5. What are different causes of mouth breathing?

Reader's Notes

14

Forces

◎ What are different types of forces?

Type of forces:

(A) **Continuous** = are those forces acting continuously without much appreciable decay. So the magnitude of the force remains constant.

- e.g. light wire appliance;
- Very light force
- Direct resorption, so no hyalinisation.
- No rest period
- *Decrease little in magnitude*

(B) **Intermittent**, e.g. removable appliance

- *Become zero with time and show the decay in b/w activations.*
    - High forces initially.
    - Require frequent activations.

(C) **Interrupted forces,** –e.g. Headgears, FA

- Heavy forces (200-300 gm).
- Used for 12-14 -hr / day.
- *Become zero abruptly when appliances are removed.*

◎ What are light orthodontic forces?

These are those forces, which are very less in magnitude and do not cause hyalinization of tissues during the OTM. Orthodontic force should be light and gentle for rapid OTM and should be 1-2 Oz. (OTM = orthodontic tooth movement).

◎ Why an adequate rest period is necessary during the active orthodontic movement?

Since with the application of the forces, the biochemical reactions start in the tissues with bone resorption, etc., a rest period is necessary for repair work of the damaged / turn-overing tissues.

◎ What are the main differences b/w orthodontic and orthopaedic forces?

Orthodontic forces	Orthopaedic forces
Light, 50-100 gm	Heavy > 400 gm/side
Continuous	Interrupted 12-14 -hr.
Dentoalveolar effects	Skeletal effects
Lead to direct resorption	Cause hyalinisation and rear resorption.

◎ What is the position of various centers of resistance related to the dentofacial complex?

C Res of single rooted tooth	In mid root region, 2/3 rd the distance from apex of the root.
C Res of molar	Bifurcation, midroot region
C Res of Maxilla Crot. For bodily OTM	Zygomatic maxillary suture at infinity
Cervical HGV causes (Head gear)	Extrusion of maxillary molars, Increase LFH
C. Res of mandibular dentition	Apical and b/w the roots of premolars.
HPHG and Kloehn HG cause	Intrusion of maxillary molars and restricts maxillary growth

◎ **What is the advantage of passing the force through the c. res. of the tooth or the unit?**

It helps in the bodily displacement of the tooth or the unit. If a force is passing at a distance from the C. Res, it leads to generation of moments and hence the rotation of the body.

◎ **Which are the main PDL fibers affected during the OTM?**

Main fibers affected during OTM and most abundant are OBLIQUE FIBRES;

◎ **What is physiological tooth movement?**

It is the movement which occurs naturally during and after the teeth eruption. Eg mesial migration of teeth, dental eruption etc.

◎ **What is the mechanism of tooth eruption?**

Dental eruption is explained by hammock ligament theory and by periodontal ligament traction theory especially the oblique fibers.

◎ **What do you mean by Squeeze film effect?**

By Bien–when very heavy forces are applied, the interstitial fluid of PDL gets squeezed out and moves towards apex and cervical margins and results in decreased OTM.

◎ **Which are the different phases of OTM?**

3 PHASES OF OTM:

Very rapid OTM	=	In Initial phase, by compression of PDL by the applied forces.
Little / no OTM	=	In lag phase, DUE TO HYALINISATION in PDL.
Rapid OTM	=	In post-lag phase, due to removal of hyalinised areas and removal of bone.

◎ **What are the various theories of OTM?**

1. Pressure–tension theory

2. Fluid dynamic theory
3. Peizoelectric theory

◎ What is piezoelectricity?

It is the phenomenon in which the deformation in the crystal structure leads to a flow of electric current due to displacement of electrons. It has 2 features, i.e. quick decay rate and after release of force, the current flows in the opposite direction.

Concave areas in bone have negative charges and lead to bone deposition. Convex areas have positive charges and bone resorption occurs.

◎ Which are the first and second messengers in OTM?

First messengers in OTM = PTH, PG, Subs P, VIP

2nd messengers in OTM= CAMP, CGMP, Ca^{2+}

◎ Where lie the areas of pressure and tension in the PDL during the tipping and bodily movements of the tooth?

During tipping = areas of pressure lie at the alveolar crest in the direction of the applied force, and at the apical area in the opposite side.

Areas of tension lie at the apical area in the direction opposite to the force applied and at the alveolar crest in opposite side.

During bodily movement = the area of pressure lies along full length of PDL in the force direction, while area of tension is along the full length of PDL on the opposite side.

◎ Why the osteoid bone is more resistant to resorption?

It is organic, uncalcified and acellular material. So it acts as a protective covering on the bone being resorbed under the forces.

◎ Which periodontal tissue is called as the slave of the orthodontist?

Alveolar bone.

◎ How much force is required for different type of tooth movements?

Forces required for tooth movements:

1. Tipping	-	50-75 gm
2. Bodily movement	-	100-150 gm
3. Intrusion	-	15-25 gm
4. Extrusion	-	50-75 gm
5. Torquing	-	50-75 gm
6. Uprighting	-	75-125 gm
7. Rotation	-	50-75 gm
8. Head Gears	-	350-450 gms on each side for a minimum of 12-14 hr / day
9. Face mask	-	1 pound (450 gm) per side, (12-14 hr),
10. Chin cup	-	Initially 150-300 gm / side; increased to 450-700 gm per side (for 12-14 hr.)

◎ What do you mean by optimal force?

Optimal force = It is the force which moves the teeth most rapidly and causes no damage to tooth and associated tissues; and with minimum patient discomfort. It is equivalent to capillary blood pressure. It amounts to 20–26 gm / cm^2 of the root surface area. It is also ka Oppenheim's philosophy.

◎ What are the 4 degrees/levels of the forces according to Schwarz?

1. First degree = force which is too gentle or of too short duration to produce any tooth movement.
2. Second degree = is the ideal force; it produces the OTM without the tissue damage.
3. Third degree = force which exceeds capillary blood pressure and could produce damage; but it is reversible if pressure is removed.
4. Fourth degree = force which produces irreversible damage in the investing tissues. It is followed by strangulation of apical vessels and death of the pulp.

◎ **What is the rate of OTM?**

Under optimal forces, it should not be > 1 mm / month.

◎ **What is the role of PD membrane?**

It acts as protective cushion; source of nutrients; storehouse of the cells and the sensory plexus.

◎ **How much time is required for the rearrangement of PD fibres and the gingival fibres?**

PDL fibers require 28 days and the gingival fibres require approx 232 days for rearranging themselves.

It is due to this slow reorganization of trans-septal/supra-alveolar tissues that the correction of rotation should be retained for a longer time.

◎ **What is the value of an ounce and a pound?**

An ounce is 28.6 gms, And a pound is 453.9 gms.

◎ **What is the value of an inch?**

It is 2.54 cm in one inch; or roughly 25.4 mm in an inch.

◎ **What is frontal resorption and the undermining/rear resorption?**

When the lighter orthodontic forces are applied, there is compression of PDL on the pressure side. The bone resorption there is seen in the alveolar bone immediately adjacent to the ligament. It is ka frontal resorption.

Rear resorption is seen when the forces applied are heavy and cause crushing of the PDL. It leads to hyalinization of the PDL and so bone resorption cannot occur there. Hence the bone resorption occurs in adjacent marrow spaces and in the alveolar plate above, below and behind the areas of hyalinization.

◎ **What are the types of root resorption?**

It is of 3 types:

1. Micro-resorption = is confined to cementum; is localised, superficial, and gets repaired.

2. Progressive root resorption= appears at the site of continuous and heavy forces; it may involve entire apex.
3. Idiopathic root resorption = it is seen even before the start of orthodontic treatment. It gets aggravated by the orthodontic treatment.

◎ Which is the most common root resorption index used?

1. Grade I = irregular root contour
2. Grade II = root resorption at the apex; is < 2 mm.
3. Grade III = root resorption from 2 mm to 1/3rd of the root length.
4. Grade IV = root resorption is > 1/3rd of the root length.

◎ What should be quality of the orthodontic force for best results?

It should be light continuous force leading to a healthy response of the tissues, without causing damage to the tissues.

◎ What change in the pattern of trabeculae is seen during the orthodontic movement of the tooth?

Normally trabeculae are parallel to the long axis of the teeth as to provide best support to them and direct the occlusal forces along and parallel to the long axis of the teeth.

With the application of the forces, the trabeculae become horizontally oriented, i.e. parallel to the direction of the orthodontic forces. However, this pattern reverses back to normal during the retention phase.

◎ What is the pitch of the expansion screw?

Pitch of the screw is the amount of opening achieved with a full turn, i.e. 360 degrees opening of the screw. Usually, it is 0.8 mm. So with each 90 degree, i.e. 1/4th turn activation of the screw, 0.2 mm (0.1 mm / side) opening occurs. Since the width of PDL is 0.22 mm, this tissue is not crushed and remains viable.

◎ **What do you mean by center of resistance, and the center of rotation?**

C. Res is the point on the tooth, through which if a force is passed, it causes the bodily movement of the tooth. In a single rooted tooth, it lies b/w 1/3rd and ½ of the root. But in a multirooted tooth, it lies b/w the roots about 1–2 mm apical to furcation.

C. res of maxillary dental arch lies in b/w the premolar roots near the apices; C. res of maxilla lies in the area of zygomaticomaxillary suture.

C. rot, is a point around a body appears to rotate when a force is applied.

C. rot of the bodily movement lies at the infinity.

C. rot. During pure rotation coincides with the C. res of the tooth.

◎ **Which all tooth movements can be carried out?**

There are 3 basic tooth movements, i.e. tipping, translation and rotation. However, the movements which are carried out are: tipping, translation, intrusion, extrusion, torquing, uprighting.

◎ **What is tipping and its types?**

It is the simplest tooth movement, requires light forces; crown moves in one direction and the root moves in the other direction.

It can be controlled tipping and the uncontrolled tipping.

Controlled tipping = the tooth tips about the c. rot at the apex. In torquing, the c. rot lies at the incisal edge, in which lingual movement of the root occurs.

Uncontrolled tipping = i.e. c. rot lies in the mid-root area, and so the crown and the root move in opposite directions.

◎ **How much force is achieved during expansion?**

Forces in expansion - SME = 2-4 lbs
- RME = 10-20 lbs

◎ What is the amount of minimum force to be applied to cause tooth movement?

It is 7 gm/cm^2.

◎ What is the minimum time for which force should be applied to cause tooth movement?

The force should be applied continuously for at least 6 hours to effect the tissue reactions.

◎ What is the direction of force application by reverse head gear / Delaire's face mask?

It is used for the correction of maxillary deficiency. D and F pull of headgear force (15–20° to OP) is applied (450 gm/side for 12-14 -hr/ day. The best age is approx. 8 yrs age to attain the skeletal effects, because it is the time of maximum maxillary growth. The force is applied in the region of primary molars so that the force may be directed through' the Cres. Of maxillary bone for maximum skeletal effects.

◎ Why are the light forces preferred over the heavy forces during orthodontic movement?

Light continuous forces are better and preferred as they cause **frontal resorption.** Heavy forces cause **rear resorption / undermining resorption** and are damaging to the investing tissues.

◎ Why the lowest amount of force is required during intrusion, although it is considered a very difficult movement?

Pressure is measured as the force per unit area. As the forces are distributed in very small periapical area during intrusion, leading to heavy pressure (P = force per unit area). So light forces lead to less pressure and so the health of PA tissues and vitality is maintained.

◎ Why the NSAIDs drugs are to be avoided during OTM?

PGE1 plays an important role in OTM (Arachidonic acid metabolites).

NSAIDS, i.e. Brufen, etc. inhibit OTM as they interfere with production of prostaglandins. Nimesulide does not interfere with PG production and so can be safely given during OTM.

◎ **What are the different CHARACTERISTICS OF WIRES?**

Longer / thinner wires decrease the load-deflection rate and provide a more gentle force system. Also, force decay is less.

STRENGTH = STIFFNESS × RANGE.
$D^3/L = D^4/L^3 \times L^2/D$
SPRINGINESS = 1/ STIFFNESS

◎ **What is the role of incorporating the loops and helices in the wire?**

Loops / helices are given in wire – to increase wire length and so to decrease the forces applied (lighter) and decrease LDR, increase the range of action.

Force is directly proportional to D^4 / L^3, thus the long lever arm reduces the force.

◎ **What is the load–deflection rate of the wires?**

It is the property according to which, how much distance a wire can be deflected on application of load without permanent deformation. If same force causes more deflection in one wire than the other wire, the former wire will apply less force for a unit deflection and also the force decay will be slower in it.

◎ **Which wire has got the property of shape memory and pseudo-elasticity?**

Ni–Ti wires.

◎ **Which is the hardest wire among these, i.e. S.S, Ni Ti, TMA and elgiloy?**

The hardest wire is S.S.

◎ **What are the different types of springs?**

1. Open coil springs and closed coil springs = s.s, Ni-Ti. They are used with fixed appliances only.

2. Simple / compound; helical / looped; self supported / supported; buccal / palatal etc.

◎ **What is the role of heat treatment for stainless steel (s.s) wires?**

It helps to remove the stresses incorporated in the wire due to manipulation of the wire and hence the slippage at the grain boundaries. It makes the formed wire harder. The wire should be heated up to straw–color only. If wire becomes red–hot during heating, it looses its properties and becomes dead.

◎ **Why do we incorporate helices, loops etc. in the wires?**

These features increase the total length of the wire and so make the structure more flexible and so applies lighter forces to the tooth.

◎ **In which direction should the helix should be activated to get the best results?**

The helices should get closed during activation, e.g. in finger spring, the helix is bent in a direction opposite to the direction of tooth movement.

Self Assessment Questions

1. What is a headgear?
2. What are the types of headgear?
3. Springs for tooth movement should be made in which wire?
4. Define Force?
5. How does the length of wire affect the forces and the tooth movement?
6. Define center of resistance and center of rotation?

Reader's Notes

15

Anchorage

◎ **Define anchorage?**

It is the nature and degree of resistance to displacement as offered by an anatomic unit for effecting a tooth movement.

◎ **Classify anchorage; and define simple, stationary, reciprocal, single, compound, multiple / reinforced, inter maxillary/ intra maxillary; intraoral; extraoral; muscular and cortical anchorages.**

Simple	-	Resistance to tipping
Stationary	-	Resistance to bodily OTM
Reciprocal	-	Tooth move equal and opposite
Minimum	-	> ½ extraction space can be lost by mesial movement of the anchor teeth.
Moderate	-	¼ to ½ extraction space can be lost by mesial movement of the anchor teeth.
Maximum	-	< ¼ extraction space can be lost by mesial movement of the anchor teeth.
Hammock	-	By PDL
Muscular	-	By lower lip, e.g. lip bumper, etc.
Cortical	-	By mandibular cortex (Rickett's)

Extraoral Anchorage = Which is obtained by sources outside the oral cavity, e.g. head gear.

Intraoral Anchorage	=	Elastics, TPA, LHA, NPA, More number of teeth involved
Baker's Anchorage	=	Class II, III elastics
Single /primary anchorage	=	Only one tooth acts as anchorage
Compound anchorage	=	More than one tooth acts as anchorage
Reinforced / multiple anchorage	=	Where more than one type of resistance unit is used.

Anchorage loss is more in maxilla than mandible, due to more cancellous bone in maxilla.

Mandibular teeth provide better anchorage than maxillary teeth due to dense bone and direction of trabeculae.

Triangular roots of canines and maxillary incisors offer maximum resistance to displacement than the round / flat roots.

◎ Why it is not possible to move the ankylosed teeth?

Because for a tooth to move, a viable PDL is required so that the biochemical changes can take place. In an ankylosed tooth, a part of PDL gets fused with the bone and so a tooth cannot move.

◎ How does the implant serve as the anchorage source?

Implant does not have any PDL, but gets engaged with the bone through osseo-integration, similar to an ankylosed tooth and so they cannot move even under heavy force, so the implants are very good anchorage.

◎ What do you mean by muscular anchorage?

Perioral ms can be used as a source of anchorage for effecting the movement of teeth, eg lip bumper uses force of lower lips to distalize or to upright the lower molars.

◎ What is Baker's anchorage?

When anchorage of one arch is used to cause movement in the opposite arch, it is ka Baker's anchorage. Eg class II, and III intermaxillary elastics.

◎ What is meant by the cortical anchorage?

According to Rickettes, when the roots of lower molars are torqued in the buccal cortical plate of mandible under heavy forces, there occurs the hyalinization of PDL, which does not allow the mesial movement or the loss of anchorage due to heavy cortical bone. It acts as the cortical anchorage.

◎ What is the anchorage loss?

It is the unwanted movement of the anchor teeth during the orthodontic treatment. It is observed by mesial tilting of the molars, labial movement of the incisors, etc.

◎ What are the anchorage savers?

These are the modalities applied during treatment so as to avoid the loss of anchorage under the forces, e.g. Head Gear, Trans-Palatal Arch, Lingual Holding Arch, Nance Palatal Arch, etc.

Self Assessment Questions

1. What are the signs of anchorage loss?
2. What are the anchorage values as provided by the upper and lower teeth?
3. What do you mean by Group A, B and C anchorage?
4. What do you mean by extraoral anchorage?
5. How do you obtain anchorage in treatment a removable appliance?
6. What factors/methods can be used for preserving the anchorage during orthodontic treatment?

Reader's Notes

16

Expansion

◎ **What are the various appliances for the fixed expansion procedure?**

Fixed Expansion by–Coffin, Haas, Hyrex, quad helix, w-arch, bihelix, NPE

◎ **What are the main differences between RME and SME?**

	RME	**SME**
1. Opening	0.5-1 mm / day (3.5–7 mm / week) 90° BD	1 mm/week 90° / 2-3 days
2. Force generated	10-20 lbs	2-4 lbs
3. Tissue damage	More	Less
4. Skeletal : dental expansion.	8:2	5:5
5. After 4 months of retention	5:5	5:5

◎ **Which of the above-said procedures are considered better, i.e. RME or SME?**

SME is definitely better as seen from the above table, because the end-result of both the procedures is the same, i.e. 1:1 achievement of dental and the skeletal effects. But SME forces are within the safe and physiological limits and comfortable to the patient.

◎ What is the pitch of the E-screw?

It is the amount of opening achieved with full one turn / 360 degrees of the E–screw. It is approx 0.8 mm. So with 90 degrees turn, we achieve the 0.2 mm opening of the screw, i.e. 0.1 mm / side of the arch.

◎ What is the width of PDL?

Normal width of PDL is approx 0.22–0.25 mm. So with 90 degree opening, only 0.1 mm / side of the PDL is compressed and so the health of the tissues is maintained under light forces.

◎ Which of the following is better–SME or RME and why?

SME is better than the RME except under exceptional circumstances. It is because, SME applies the forces with in the physiological range without damaging the investing tissues.

◎ How much space can be gained by expansion?

If we consider the upper arch as half circle till the first molar region, we can gain a space approx 1.56 mm / mm of expansion.

◎ What modalities are available for expansion?

Coffin spring, porter's appliance, bihelix, quad-helix appliance, NPE, i.e. Ni-Ti palatal expanders, fixed expansion appliance, TPA, etc. besides removable jackscrew appliances.

◎ Why this name has been given to the quad helix appliance?

It contains 4 helices in the design so it is called by this name.

◎ Why Coffin appliance is called so?

It was first designed by Coffin.

◎ What is the role of the helices in the quad helix appliance?

Helices increase the length of the wire in the appliance. So lighter forces are applied by the appliance.

◎ What is the advantage of Ni-Ti palatal expanders?

Since it keeps on applying a light continuous force on the tissues, it is tissue-friendly. Also there is no need of repeated removal of this appliance for activation as the Ni-Ti wire has shape memory property.

◎ What are the main contraindications of expansion?

It is not indicated in vertical growth pattern cases, as it tends to worsen the facial pattern. Also, it is not indicated in the patient who are past their growth age.

◎ How does the expansion improve the respiration pattern?

It increases the area of nasal passage and so reduces the resistance to air flow. So the pattern can change from mouth to nasal pattern

◎ What are the other uses of E–screw?

It can be used

- for distalization of molar to gain space;
- to move the incisors anteriorly in case of Class II div 2 m.o;
- to gain space for correction of cross bite of maxillary canine;
- to expand arches in CLP patients;
- to widen the arches in case of treatment with myofunctional appliances in Class II div 1 m.o.

◎ Till what age, the mid-palatal suture is not ossified?

It ossifies at approx 12–14 yrs of age. After this, only dental effects come in effect with least skeletal effect with expansion.

◎ Till what age, the skeletal effects can be gained by expansion?

Most of the skeletal effects can be achieved at approx 8–9 yrs of the age, however decrease amounts of skeletal effects are still achievable till 12–14 yrs age.

◎ What is the pattern of expansion?

Opening of the mid-palatal suture is fan-shaped, i.e. maximum opening at the incisor region decreasing progressively posteriorly. Similarly, it is there in the superio-inferior direction, with maximum opening towards the oral cavity. Also, with expansion, maxilla rotates in a downward and forward direction. So it helps in correcting the maxillary hypoplasia. It is also indicated before starting the Delaire's face mask therapy. It leads to proclination of maxillary incisors.

◎ What is the best age for expansion and why?

8–9 yrs is the best age for expansion, as it is an approx time for a growth spurt to come and also, the mid-palatal suture is also viable and not interdigitated.

◎ If a patient of 25 yrs age comes to you with narrow maxillary arch indicated for expansion, what will you do?

Palatal expansion with surgical splitting will be done.

◎ What is the difference b/w arch expansion and arch augmentation?

Arch expansion is the widening the arch in the transverse direction, while the arch augmentation is the lengthening the arch by moving the teeth in anterior / labial direction eg in Class II div 2 cases.

Self Assessment Questions

1. Why expansion is contraindicated in vertical growth pattern cases?
2. Till what relationship of upper and lower cusps, the expansion should be done during R_x?
3. Why overexpansion is done while expanding and till what limit?
4. Which analyses/indices give indication for requirement of expansion in a particular case?
5. What are the chances of stable results in expanded mandibular arch?
6. How does mandibular intercanine width affect the expansion decision in mandibular arch?
7. Why there are great chances of relapse of expansion in a surgically treated case of cleft palate?
8. What is the advantage of posterior bite plane in expansion appliances in case of vertical growth pattern?
9. What is Porter's appliance?

Reader's Notes

17

Extractions

◎ **What are the different extraction procedures undertaken in orthodontics?**

- **Wilkinson's extraction** = Removal of all first permanent molars, at 8½–9 ½ years age
- **Stobie's extraction** = removal of ADJACENT premolars at one time.
- **Therapeutic extraction** = Removal of teeth for treatment–purpose.
- **Balancing** = Removal of teeth from both sides in same arch
- **Compensating** = Removal of teeth from same side in both arches.
- **Serial extraction** = removal of CD4
- Serial extraction procedures are usually related to the eruption pattern of permanent mandibular 3,4.

◎ **What are the disadvantages of serial extraction?**

Serial extraction causes **deepening of bite**, due to lingual inclination and uprighting of lower incisors. It always requires a second phase of orthodontic treatment by fixed orthodontic appliance.

◎ **What are the indications of extraction of second premolars during the fixed orthodontic treatment?**

Main indication of second premolar extraction especially in the mandibular arch, is that the discrepancy should be present in the mid-arch segment; the incisors should be well aligned without any appreciable or with very mild crowding. It is mainly indicated for the correction of end-on molar relationship to class I molar by loosing anchorage in lower arch.

◎ What are the disadvantages of second premolar extraction?

Main side effect of second PM extraction is the deepening of bite, due to mesial molar movement and so overclosure / autorotation of the mandible. So, it should be avoided in the horizontal growing cases especially Class II div 2 cases.

◎ What is the side effect of lower incisor extraction?

Single extraction of lower incisor leads to narrowing of the lower intercanine width. But since the intercanine width of upper arch is the same, this may lead to appearance of crowding in the upper anterior segment.

Self Assessment Questions

1. Which analyses help us to determine the requirement of extractions during treatment planning?
2. In which cases the extractions of permanent first molars is indicated?
3. What is the effect of extraction treatment on the over bite?
4. What is Angle's concept regarding extractions and R_x-planning?
5. What is the latest terminology of serial extraction known as?
6. What are the indications of serial extraction?
7. What are the indications of canine extraction?

Reader's Notes

18

Orthodontic Appliances

◎ **What is a removable appliance?**

The appliance which can be removed by the patient for cleaning etc.

◎ **What is a fixed appliance?**

An appliance which cannot be removed by the patient, but can be removed by the doctor only.

◎ **What is a mechanical appliance?**

Appliances which can apply pressure on teeth and the supporting tissues for the purpose of tooth movement by the active components.

◎ **What is a myofunctional appliance?**

These are the appliances which derive their force from the muscles for the correction of teeth and the jaw relationship.

◎ **What is a semi-fixed appliance?**

These are the appliances, a part of which can be removed by the patient but not the whole appliance.

◎ **What is an active appliance?**

These are the appliances which can exert the forces by their active components for effecting the tooth movement.

◎ **What is a passive appliance?**

These appliances does not apply forces on the teeth and their investing tissues. These are given as adjunctive modalities during the active treatment.

◎ **What is a retention appliance?**

These are the appliances, which are passive in nature, and are used to maintain the positions of the corrected teeth in their new locations after the orthodontic treatment is over. So they function to avoid the relapse. All retentive appliances are passive in nature, but all passive appliances are not retentive.

◎ **What is a tooth borne appliance?**

It is the appliance which is totally supported by the teeth.

◎ **What is a tissue borne appliance?**

This is the appliance which derives its support from the soft tissues surrounding the teeth.

◎ **What is a tooth–tissue borne appliance?**

These appliances derive the support from both the teeth and the tissues.

◎ **What is a myotonic appliance?**

Myofunctional appliances which depend on their muscle mass for their action.

◎ **What is a myodynamic appliance?**

Myofunctional appliances which depend on the muscles activity for their action.

◎ **What is an orthopaedic appliance?**

An appliance which applies heavy forces for the purpose of causing changes in the skeletal relations of the jaw bases.

◎ **What is an orthodontic appliance?**

An appliance which applies lighter forces for causing the movement of teeth in the alveolar bone, without causing any skeletal changes.

◎ **What do you mean by group I myofunctional appliance?**

These appliances transfer their forces directly to the teeth for correction of malocclusion.

◎ What do you mean by group II myofunctional appliance?

Appliances reposition the mandibular base and the resulting forces are then transmitted to the teeth and the supporting tissues for correction of malocclusion.

◎ What do you mean by group III myofunctional appliance?

These appliances also cause repositioning of the mandible, but their area of operation is vestibule of the mouth, e.g. Frankel appliance.

◎ What are the basic components of a removable appliance and their functions?

There are 3 basic parts, i.e. retentive components, active components and acrylic base plate.

Retentive components = help in retaining the appliance in place.

Active components = help in applying forces for the movement of the teeth.

Base plate = binds all the components into a single functional unit.

◎ What are the various active components?

These are labial bows, springs, screws and elastics.

Labial bows are = short and long labial bows; split labial bow; reverse labial bow; high labial bow with apron spring; fitted labial bow; Robert's retractor and Mill's retractor.

Active labial bows are generally made in 22 or 23 gauge s.s wire.

Passive / retentive bows are made in 21 gauge s.s wires.

Bows used in functional appliances are made in 19 or 20 gauge s.s wires.

Springs can be = simple/ compound; helical / looped; self-supported / supported springs.

◎ Which are the factors on which the flexibility of the spring depends?

It depends directly on the cube of the length of the wire; inversely on the fourth power of the diameter of the wire (D^4/L^3).

◎ What is the load–deflection rate of a wire?

It signifies the flexibility of the wire. It means the amount of the deflection of the wire under a specific load. If we compare 2 wires of different length and / or diameter, the thinner wire / longer wire is deflected more than the other one under the same load and hence it applies less force under the same distance of activation. It also signifies the loss of force / force–decay during the tooth movement for the amount of the deflection of the wire. A low L–D rate is required for the active orthodontic appliance.

◎ What are various retentive components?

These are Adams clasp; pin head; C–clasp; southend clasp; crozat clasp; Jackson's clasp; triangular clasp; ball–end clasp, etc.

◎ What are the various common appliances used in the orthodontics with their main functions?

Coffin Spring	Expansion
Quad helix	Expansion
Jack screw	Expansion
Porter (W-arch)	Expansion
Bihelix	Expansion
Schwarz App	Expansion
NPE I, II	Expansion
TPA, LHA, NPA	Space maintenance, anchorage savers
Distal shoe appliance; aka Roche's appliance	For guiding mandibular Permanent first molar to erupt after premature loss of primary mandibular first molar
Anterior bite plate	Bite opening
Posterior bite plate with z-spring	Treatment of anterior cross bite
Reverse bite plate	Bite opening and mandibular forward displacement

Catalan's/(L) inclined plane	Treatment of anterior cross bite
Bionater, Twin-block	Myofunctional
Activator, FR etc.	Myofunctional
Herbst, Jasper Jumper	Myofunctional, fixed
Chin cup, Petit's/ and Hickham appliance, Delaire's face mask	For treatment of Skeletal Class III
Oral screen	For treatment of protruded incisors with spacing, and for expansion of arches
Cetlin appliance, pendulum app., distal jet	Molar distalisation
Lip bumber	For hyperactive mentalis m, lip sucking; anchorage
Tongue blade	Treatment of Anterior cross bite
M-spring	Closure of midline diastema
Hewley's appliance	For retention (also known as DENTAL CRUTCH)
Clip on retainer	For retention
Kesling tooth positioner	For retention
Nakamura's	Treatment of class III
Jackson's Clasp	U-shaped
¾ circumferential	C- shaped
Southend Clasp	M- shaped (anterior region)
Triangular clasp	
Ball-end clasp	
Schwarz clasp	Also known as Arrow Head Clasp with a number of arrow heads
Crozat Pin head	U-shaped with wire soldered

- Finger spring–for MD OTM
- Z spring–for labial OTM
- T- spring, paddle/ flapper for labial OTM
- M spring = closure of midline diastema

◎ Which is the most basic removable appliance?

Hawley's appliance is the most basic removable appliance and so other appliances are the modification of this appliance. It is known as dental crutch also. It is a passive appliance. The main purpose of this appliance is the retention.

◎ Which appliance is used for the mesiodistal movement of the teeth?

A removable appliance with *finger–spring* incorporated in the appliance is used. This helps to close the diastema b/w the teeth. The finger spring is made of 22 or 23 gauge s.s. wire.

◎ What are various features of a finger spring?

1. The active arm touches the tooth.
2. The helix is made in the direction opposite to the direction of the tooth movement. Helix helps to generate the light forces. A rule of thumb is that the helix should close on activation for application of the proper force.
3. The helix is placed generally midway b/w the initial and the final position of the tooth.
4. Internal diameter of the helix is 3 times the diameter of the wire.
5. Helix is placed at least 5 mm beyond the free gingival margin, near to the c. res of the tooth, and it should be parallel to the palatal surface.
6. The active arm should be placed towards the palatal tissues.
7. The activation should be approx 3 mm, such that it is able to produce a movement @ 1 mm / month.

8. The length of the retentive arm should be longer than the active by at least 1.5 times.
9. The retentive arm should not cross the midline.

◎ Which appliance is used for the labial movement of the tooth?

Various components can be used eg Z–spring; E–screw; paddle spring and T–spring. It is generally used for the treatment of the cross–bite relation of the incisors and / or tooth in linguoversion, eg in Class II div 2 cases.

A posterior bite plane is incorporated in the appliance to create a gap b/w the incisal edges.

Z–spring is made of 22 or 23 gauge wire. It is made with 2 helices; the active arm should be towards the apex of the tooth and force applied by this spring is perpendicular to the long axis of the tooth.

◎ What is the prerequisite for the alignment of any tooth in the arch?

Adequate space should be present / created for the proper alignment of the tooth in the arch, e.g. during the treatment of cross bite; during the retraction of the incisors, etc.

◎ Which appliance is used for the lingual movement of the teeth?

Mostly, labial bow is used for this purpose. The bow is made active, in 22 or 23 gauge wire. The level is generally placed at the junction of incisal and the middle 3rd of the crown. It should be parallel to the incisal edges of the anterior teeth. The length of the U–loop should be such that it should extend only 2 mm below the free marginal gingiva of the canine.

◎ What is the main disadvantage of the removable appliance?

It causes the tipping of the tooth, eg with crown moving lingually, the root moves labially.

Also, only simple tooth movements can be done.

The success rate depends on the cooperation of the patient.

Finishing of teeth positioning is poor.

◎ What is the role of the canine retractors?

It helps to move the labially / mesially erupted canines in the arch. If space is not there, it is created by removal of first premolar.

Disadvantage of this appliance is the mesio-labial rotation of the canine, due to the force being applied labial to the center of rotation of the tooth.

◎ What is an anterior bite plate appliance?

- It is a modified Hawley's appliance, which has got a ramp extending from canine to canine in maxillary arch appliance.
- It is used for opening of deep bite; it is best in average / horizontal growth pattern cases;

◎ Why it is contraindicated in vertical growth pattern cases?

- C/I in vertical growth cases since with the eruption of molars, the mandible moves in a downward and backward direction, which further increases facial height and profile becomes more convex.

◎ What is the mechanism of action of anterior bite plate?

- It mechanism of action is that it allows the supra-eruption of mandibular molars for opening of the deep bite.
- 2-3 mm inter-occlusal gap in the first molar region is created for supra-eruption of mandibular molars. The plane of the plate is kept parallel to the OP.
- Further opening of the bite can be accomplished step–wise.

◎ If the inter-occlusal gap is more than 2–3 mm, what problem can be encountered with anterior bite plate?

If gap is > 4-5 mm = Tongue interferes with molar eruption and bite does not correct

◎ What is the side effect of anterior bite plate appliance?

Causes anterior force on (U) incisors leading to flaring of these teeth. So it is good for C_2D_2 m.o.

◎ What is deep bite and how it is classified?

It is the vertical overlap of upper incisors to the lower incisors more than the normal, i.e. 2 mm. It can be classified as skeletal / dental; complete / incomplete, etc.

◎ How can we treat a deep bite case?

It depends on the growth pattern of the patient; and upper lip relation of the incisors. In case of horizontal growth pattern, the molar extrusion should be done for it, as it leads to the down and back rotation of the mandible. But in case of vertical growth pattern, the molar extrusion should not be done, as it may deteriorate the facial profile and increase the face height.

Also, if upper lip length is normal but there is gummy smile or increased visibility of upper incisors, the upper incisors should be intruded.

◎ What is the normal relationship of upper lip to the incisal edges of upper teeth?

At rest, the incisal edges of upper incisors are exposed by only 2–3 mm.

◎ What is the normal relationship of upper lip to the upper teeth in full smile?

If the length of upper lip is normal with the normal inclination of upper incisors, the upper lip in full smile lies at the level of the gingival margin of the upper incisors.

◎ What is a reverse bite plate appliance?

It is modified Hawley's appliance which has got a ramp extending from canine to canine, but its plane is kept at 45–60 degrees angle to the OP.

◎ What are the indications of this appliance?

It is mainly used for the opening of the bite; and brings the mandible forward in cases of the mandibular retrognathism cases. It is best used during the growth phase of the child.

◎ **What is the mechanism of action of this appliance?**

It helps to open the bite; it also shifts the mandible forward along the incline especially in Class II div 1 cases; as the plane is kept at 45–60 degrees to OP. Interocclusal gap should be 2–3 mm in the first molar region.

◎ **What is the side effect of this appliance?**

It causes an anterior force on (L) incisors and hence their flaring, as the mandible, which has been slid forward on the ramp tries to go back to its original position under the influence of its attached ms.

◎ **What is a posterior bite plate appliance?**

It is a modified Hawley's appliance, either in upper or lower arch, having acrylic covering the occlusal surfaces of the posterior teeth, so that the teeth of the opposing arch are in even contact with it.

◎ **What is the use of this appliance?**

- It helps to create a gap between incisal edges of U/L teeth, i.e. incisal clearance during the treatment of anterior cross bite with the help of Z–springs, etc.
- It also helps to treat the anterior open bite by causing intrusive forces on the molars.
- It also helps to create a gap b/w the occlusal surfaces of one side of the teeth, if the other side is in cross bite and needs expansion of the arch.

◎ **What precaution should be taken while making such appliance?**

- All the posterior teeth should be touching the acrylic ramp evenly on both the sides for efficient mastication.
- The height of the acrylic should not be excessive as it may lead to fatigue of the ms of mandible.

◎ **How it is helpful during the expansion therapy in cases of vertical growth pattern cases?**

It is used in the expansion appliances to avoid the extrusion of the molars during expansion in such cases.

◎ **What are the important features of a HAWLEY'S Retention appliance?**

- Is the most basic of the removable appliance.
- It contains Adams clasps, labial bow and the acrylic base plate.
- The acrylic should be touching all the teeth of that arch on the lingual surfaces just above their height of contour / HOC. It helps to avoid the movement / relapse of the teeth on lingual side / or of rotations.
- Labial bow should be made *passive*, made in 21 or 20 gauge S.S. wire; should be evenly touching the teeth to avoid their labial displacement.
- *Level of the labial bow* should be in the middle of the crown of the teeth. It helps to avoid the relapse of the torque corrections.
- Can be modified with cribs in case of habits and in other cases.

◎ **What is a Habit breaking appliance?**

- Used for those patients who themselves want to leave the habit.
- These are *not the punishment appliances* but the reminder appliances.
- Main component is the cribs made of 21 gauge s.s wire.
- Cribs are made on the lingual side of the maxillary anterior teeth in the canine to canine region, their height adjusted so that they do not injure the lingual tissues of lower arch when mouth is closed; and also does not allow the anterior movement of the tongue or easy entry of finger in the mouth.
- The levels of the cribs should be the same, parallel to the incisal plane, and should be 1–2 mm beyond the incisal edges of maxillary incisors. It should not injure the lingual tissue of mandible.

- Position of the cribs = are usually placed in line with the lingual embrasures of upper teeth.
- Help to *break the seal* of the finger with the tongue, lips and cheeks during the digit sucking habit, and does not allow the build up of the vacuum, and so does not give the psychological satisfaction to the child.

◎ What is an Expansion appliance?

It is a modified Hawley's appliance, which has got an expansion screw place in the midline. It is use to increase the transverse dimensions of the arch. It is a very good appliance for the interception of the malocclusion.

◎ What is the position of the E-screw, and why?

- E–screw placed on the line joining the upper canines, so that force of the expansion is mainly directed in this area.
- It is because the main narrowing of the arch occurs in this area because 8 ms are attached at the corner of the mouth / modiolus, which overlies the upper canine area. When the balance of intraoral and extraoral ms is disturbed, the arch narrowing mainly occurs in this region. Similarly, in CLP cases, the main narrowing is in this region only, with the intermolar width being normal.

◎ What are the other uses of E-screw?

- It can be used to gain space during the teeth alignment; it helps to increase the nasal passage area and so in the treatment of the mouth breathing habit.
- It acts as a reminder also to a patient of digit sucking habit.
- It can be used to treat the anterior cross bite if more teeth are involved or if maxillary canine is involved. Maxillary canine being a strong tooth and having the longest root, is least affected by Z –spring.
- It is also used to labially incline the central incisors in cases of class II div 2 pattern.

◎ **What is an Oral screen / vestibular screen?**

It is an appliance which is placed in the labial vestibule of the mouth, i.e. b/w labial surfaces of the teeth inside and the lips and cheeks on outside.

◎ **Why is it known as the vestibular screen?**

Because it occupies the vestibule of the mouth.

◎ **What is the extension limit of oral screen?**

It extends posteriorly covering the mesial half of the last erupted molars, i.e. the mesial half of the maxillary first molar if given in the age range given below.

◎ **Which is the best age for the use of oral screen?**

Best age = early Mixed Dentition Period, i.e. 8-9 years, as it is the time of palatal width increase.

◎ **How does it help in expansion of the upper and lower arches?**

It helps in the expansion of arches, when spacer of wax is placed during fabrication of this appliance, extending from the canine to last molar region. Expansion occurs with the help of the tongue pressure.

◎ **What are the other uses of oral screen?**

- Retraction of upper anterior teeth, by the help of the lip forces.
- Treatment of mouth breathing, tongue thrusting; digit sucking habits.

◎ **What is the use of ring and where it is kept?**

It is kept at the junction of middle and incisal 3rd of upper C.I. (which is the normal level of the lower lip), Used for lip exercises. It should be made of 20 gauge or thicker S.S. hard wire.

◎ **What is the use of spacer placed in the oral screen?**

- Spacer provides space for expansion of arches by tongue pressure
- Modified with holes, cribs, lingual screen etc. for specific purposes.

◎ What is an inclined plane appliance?

- It is an appliance having an acrylic covering the lower incisors at an angle to the occlusal plane and touching the lingual surface/s of the upper incisors. It is used to treat the upper incisors which are erupting in the cross bite relationship, i.e. in *developing cross bite*.
- It is not successful in treating a tooth, which has completely erupted in the cross bite.
- Proper space must be there in the arch for alignment of the tooth in cross bite.

◎ How do you obtain the anchorage for the treatment of the cross bite?

At least one tooth on each side of the culprit tooth are involved in the appliance to make the anchorage surface area more than the tooth being treated.

◎ What is the angle of the incline plane?

The angle of the incline is made at approx 45–60 degrees to the occlusal plane so that the culprit incisor slides along this incline.

◎ What is the maximum time for which it should be used and why?

It should be worn only for 2–3 weeks, as the prolonged wear may cause overeruption of molars and may lead to open bite.

◎ What is a Lip bumper appliance?

- It is a removable or fixed appliance; a sort of myofunctional appliance.
- The acrylic button is fabricated in the lower anterior vestibule.

◎ What is the mechanism of action of lip bumper?

- It helps to keep the lower lip away from lower incisors and prevents their lingual tilting. It is indicated in lip sucking habits.
- It also transfers the force of lower lip to the molars and causes their distal tipping. It helps to increase the anchorage.

◎ What should be the position of the acrylic button in this appliance?

- The acrylic button should be about 5–6 mm high. It should extend from mesial of one canine to the mesial of the other canine.
- Its acrylic button should be kept 2–3 mm away from the labial surfaces of the lower incisors. This space also allows the incisors to move labially under the tongue forces.
- The acrylic button is placed at the level of the marginal gingiva of the lower incisors region, somewhat towards the vestibule, causing a stretch of the periosteum also.

◎ What are the effects of this appliance?

- This appliance helps to *avoid lip trap*, helps labial tipping of incisors, help increase the arch length by distal tipping of molars and labial tipping of incisors; avoids the lip biting habit and controls the hyperactive lower lip and mentalis m.
- It stretches the periosteum in the lower incisor region and helps in the deposition of the bone in that region.
- Its modification in the upper vestibule is ka Denholtz appliance.
- Its other modification is Augmentor appliance, which is used to treat a case of maxillary hypoplasia. It obtains its anchorage from the lower molars.

◎ How will you treat the following conditions by removable appliances?

Anterior cross bite	Z–spring in a maxillary appliance with posterior bite plate
Posterior cross bite	Z–spring or E–screw or T–screw with anterior bite plate, to create gap
Midline diastema	Finger spring. Remove the cause also.
Generalized diastema in incisor region	Labial bow only if adequate overjet present. Acrylic has to be relieved on lingual side to provide a space for lingual movement of the teeth.

Habits	Cribs in the maxillary appliance; but is normal till 3–4 yrs of age and should not be disturbed
Mesially placed canines	By canine retractors after creating space distal to canine, eg by extraction of first premolar
Contracted arch maxillary	Expansion appliance especially during the growth period
Deep bite	By anterior bite plate to allow the posterior teeth to erupt
Open bite	By giving posterior bite plane, which does not let the posteriors to erupt; and may apply the intrusive force on them.
Lingually inclined incisors	By giving z–spring lingually to push them labially, followed by retention
Mandibular retrognathism	By myofunctional appliance if the child is in growing phase;
Maxillary retrognathism	By Delaire's face mask especially during 8 yrs age;
Mandibular prognathism	By chin cup; apply orthopedic forces; should be retained till the growth period is over till 18 yrs age.
Maxillary prognathism	By head gear to restrict forward growth of maxilla
Mouth breathing	By oral screen; also helps in expansion of the arch and lingual tipping of the upper incisors
Developing cross bite	It is due to erupting incisors when its deciduous tooth is not shed; is done by inclined plane used for 2–3 weeks only.
Ugly ducking stage	Should not be disturbed as it is a normal developmental sequelae.
Supernumerary tooth	Extraction; otherwise may lead to deflected path of eruption of other teeth and so malocclusion.

Self Assessment Questions

1. What are the various sizes of elastics available for orthodontic R_x?
2. Classify deep bite condition?
3. What is the role of RAKES in R_x of habits?
4. What are the modifications of oral screen?
5. Lip bumper appliance in upper arch is also known by what name and what are its functions?
6. What is the pitch of E-screw?
7. What are the different designs of E-screw available in market?
8. What are the differences between SME and RME?

Reader's Notes

19

Fixed Orthodontic Appliances

◎ **What are the various COMPONENTS OF FIXED APPLIANCES?**

These are the bands; brackets; buccal tubes; arch wires; elastics; hooks; ligature wires and ligature rings / modules; open and close coil springs; uprighting springs; etc.

Plastic brackets are made of	Polycarbonate
Nitinol wires contain	Ni, Ti in 55 : 45, i.e. 1:1 stoichiometric ratio
β- titanium (TMA) contain	Ti, Mo
Elgiloy contains	Co, Cr, Ni
18:8 S.S. contains	18 Cr, 8 Ni

Elastics are made of Latex rubber

Class I Elastics	Intra arch, close space and retract the teeth
Class II Elastics	Inter arch, class II molar correction, retraction of (U)- anterior
Class III Elastics	Inter arch, class III molar correction, retraction of (L) anterior

(Class II, Class III also known as Baker's anchorage)

Box Elastics	for treatment open bite
Cross elastics	for treatment posterior cross bite

Triangular and check patterns	For occlusal settling

◎ **What is the force generated by the light elastics?**

It is in the range of 2–3 oz.

◎ **Which band materials are used in the orthodontics?**

- 0.180 x 0.005 "–0.006" - for molars
- 0.150 x 0.004" - for PMs, canines
- 0.125 x 0.003" - for incisors

◎ **Which brackets are mostly used in the fixed orthodontics?**

Brackets can be metallic / plastic / ceramic; curved / flat; bondable / weldable; they act as Handle for applying the forces on the teeth.

1. **Edgewise technique** = 022 × 028",.018 × 025" slot size
- Rectangular wire is used = Two point contact, help torquing.
- Bodily tooth movement.
- High forces required, more time required.

2. **Begg's technique:**
- Buccal tube = 030"
- Only tipping movement, light forces required
- Round wire, single point contact
- Less time is taken for retraction of anterior teeth.

3. **Straight wire appliance, SWA:**
- It is a modified edgewise appliance.
- It was promoted by Andrews.
- The wire bending part has been eliminated in this technique.
- The tip and torque has been incorporated in the brackets base itself.

◎ What is an arch wire; what is its role; it is made of what material?

It is the component of the fixed appliance which is ligated to the brackets for applying the forces, etc.; it also keeps the teeth bound in one unit to act as anchorage; it can also have hooks for application of elastics, etc.

It is made of different materials, viz s.s; Ni-Ti; TMA; elgiloy, etc.

◎ What are different types of the buccal tubes?

These are round / oval / rectangular; single / double / triple; weldable/ bondable / solderable; double rectangular etc.

Sizes = 030" for Begg's appliance; 018 × 025 / 022 × 028 for edgewise and SWA technique; 045" for headgear bows.

◎ What are different types of elastics used in the treatment?

The elastics are the active components to apply the forces to the teeth. The force depends on the internal diameter of the elastic and on the thickness of the elastic. Small diameter / thicker elastics apply higher forces.

The elastics have been graded according to *color-coding* as red / blue / green / yellow / cream etc for easy identification.

The size varies as 1/8; 3/16; ¼; 5/16 and 3/8 inches also according to the diameter. The elastics are also called light / medium / heavy and extra–heavy according the force applied.

The adequate force of the elastic is applied only when it is stretched to 3 times its internal diameter. The elastics used for applying the orthopedic forces are much thicker in diameter.

◎ Self Assessment Questions

1. What is an orthopedic elastic?
2. How much force is required for orthopedic effects?
3. What is the advantage of ceramic brackets?
4. What is the disadvantage of ceramic brackets?
5. What is the advantage and main features of Ni-Ti wires?

6. What is the role of multiple loop arch wires?
7. What is the role of chromium in stainless steel?
8. What are the different types of elgiloy wires?
9. What is the role of open coil Ni-Ti spring?
10. What are the methods of planing attachments on the tooth in fixed appliances?
11. What is etching? How it is done?
12. Which cements are used for band cementation and which is the best cement and why?
13. What is mechanical interlocking as achieved by etching and bonding?
14. What do you mean by "frozen slab technique" during band cementation?
15. What do you understand by first-order, second-order and third-order bands in fixed orthodontic R_x?
16. What are the different sizes of band materials for different teeth?

Reader's Notes

20

Materials Used in Orthodontics

◎ What is orthodontic wire, i.e. a cast alloy or a wrought alloy?

Orthodontic wire are made of wrought alloys.

◎ What is the carbon content in Carbon steel?

A steel with Carbon content < 1.2 % is the carbon steel.

◎ Which are the different phases of stainless steel alloys?

There are mainly 3 phases of S.S alloy, i.e. ferrite, austenite and martensite.

Ferrite is pure Fe; has BCC structure; low solubility of C (0.02 wt %); stable up to 912 °C.

Austenite = has a FCC structure; stable up to 912–1394 °C; maximum C solubility is 2.11 %. When austenite is cooled slowly, then iron carbide (Fe_3C) is precipitated out, which gives strength of softer ferrite and austenite phase. Orthodontic wires are made of austenitic S.S.

If austenite is **cooled rapidly** / quenched = a diffusion-less transformation to BCT structure is formed , ka **martensite**; it is highly distorted, strained, very hard and brittle. It is used to make **cutting edges of the instruments**.

Ferrite	**Pure Fe**	**BCC; 912 C**
Martensite	Formed by quenching the austenite phase	BCT; brittle; used for cutting instruments
Austenite		FCC; best alloy of S.S.; formed b/w 912–1394 °C.

◎ **What do you mean by tempering?**

Martensite on heating changes to ferrite and carbides. It decreases hardness and increases toughness.

◎ **Why the steel alloy is known as Stainless steel?**

It contains Cr (12–30 %), which provides a passivating effect by Oxide film and gives resistance to tarnish /corrosion to the alloy.

◎ **What is stainless steel?**

If carbon content is < 1.2 %; and Cr is 12–30 %, it is ka stainless steel. It is stainless due to formation of a protective layer of chromium oxide on the surface of the metal.

◎ **What do you mean by 18 : 8 stainless steel?**

The S.S alloy containing 18 % chromium and 8 % nickel is 18:8 s.s.

◎ **What are the important properties of Austenitic s.s?**

- Most corrosion resistant;
- 18 % Cr + 8% Ni + 0.15 % C.
- most common for orthodontic wires/ bands
- Cold workable and increases strength.
- Ease in forming.

◎ **What do you mean by the phenomenon of SENSITISATION?**

It is due to presence of chromium. If s.s. is heated b/w 400–900 °C, the corrosion resistance is lost due to precipitation of chromium carbide (Cr_3C), which is most rapid at 650 °C. So passivating effect of Cr is lost, intergranular corrosion occurs at grain boundaries. If s.s is cold worked, carbides precipitate along the slip planes rather than at grain boundaries and so resistance to corrosion is increased eg orthodontic wires.

◎ **What do you mean by STABILISATION?**

It is the process of saving the precipitation of chromium. Titanium is added to the alloy, which gets precipitated in place of Cr. The concentration of Ti should be 6 × the concentration of carbon. Austenite s.s is susceptible to attack by solutions containing chlorine, so chloride cleansers should not be used with them.

◎ What are the basic properties of stainless steel?

- In orthodontic wires, strength and hardness may increase with decrease in diameter, because if the amount of cold working in forming the wire.
- T.S = 2100 Mpa
- Y.S = 1400 Mpa
- KHN = 600

Property of readily strain hardening is a characteristic of austenite S.S. which is mainly due to phase change from FCC to BCC.

- BCC ferrite/ martensite are ferromagnetic and austenite is nonmagnetic.

◎ What do you mean by Soldering and welding?

Soldering is the uniting the 2 parts with the help of a filler material intervening in between the two parts.

Welding is the joining the 2 parts without any other material intervening. It occurs by high heat for a very brief period, i.e. for less than the 1 / 10th of a sec., the heat should be dissipated away quickly to avoid the weld decay.

◎ What should be the temperature difference b/w parts to be joined and the solder MP?

Solder's MP should be less than that of the parts being joined by at least 50 degrees C. Generally, the fusion temperature of solder should be less than 450 °C.

◎ What do you mean by brazing?

If the fusion temperature of solder being used is more than 450 °C, the process is brazing.

◎ **What is a solder?**

It is a fusible alloy used as a filler or intermediary alloy to unite, by heating, the metals and alloys which are less fusible. It flows due to capillary action b/w the 2 parts.

◎ **What is the gap recommended b/w the parts being joined during soldering?**

Approx 0.13 to 0.3 mm.

◎ **What is the role of Sn and In added to solder?**

Sn and In are added to decrease the fusion temperature and improve solderability.

◎ **What is flux and anti-flux, and what is their role?**

Flux is a material having borax and boric acid with some fluorides. It aids in removing the ***oxide layer*** from the surface of metals being joined and increase the flow of solder on the surface of metals. Composition of flux is borax glass 55 %; boric acid 35 % and silica 10 %.

Fluorides / KF dissolve **the passivating film** of chromium for better union. It also prevents oxidation of metals being joined. It is composed of boric acid and KF in 1:1 ratio.

Anti-flux–it is used to confine the flow of the solder on the parts being joined. Mostly, graphite or lead–pencil is used to mark the area of joint before start of soldering.

◎ **What is the composition of fluoride fluxes?**

Boric acid and potassium fluoride are in 1:1 ratio.

◎ **Which zone of the flame is used while soldering?**

Reducing zone / blue zone of the flame should be used. It helps to prevent the oxidation of the parts being joined and also it is having maximum heat. The Color of the molten solder should never exceed DULL RED. Use as little heat as possible, for a least possible time to avoid carbide precipitates, loss of strength, etc.

◎ What are the 2 types of soldering?

These are : free hand soldering and investment soldering.

◎ What are the types of solder?

These are soft and hard solders.

Soft solders have low melting range of approx. 260 °C; lack corrosion resistance;

Hard solders have high melting range, have more strength and more corrosion resistant; these are the most often used in dentistry.

◎ What is the composition of gold solder and silver solders?

Component	Gold solder	Silver solder
Au	45–81 %	———
Ag	8–30	10–80
Cu	7–20	15–50
Sn	2–4	———
Zn	2–4	4–35 %
Misc	———	Sn + In

◎ What is the temperature range for orthodontic silver solders?

It is 620–665 °C.

◎ After soldering, the appliance should be immediately quenched, why?

It helps to confine the heat to the joint area and prevents the spread of the heat to adjacent parts.

◎ Why a welding joint is more susceptible to corrosion?

Weld spot is seen as nugget of the resolidified cast structure. Strength of weld joint decreases by increasing recrystallisation of wrought structures. Weld joint is susceptible to corrosion due to chromium carbide precipitates and loss of passivation.

◎ What is the principal behind the welding process?

The resistance offered by S.S. to an electric current of high value generates enough heat that the alloy is softened. The current is passed through' 2 Cu–electrodes which are approximated under pressure. The resistance of the materials being joined to the flow of current produces intense local heat and actual fusion of the overlapped materials occurs.

◎ For how much time the current is passed?

It is passed for a very short time interval, i.e. < 1 / 10th of a second; so a timer is fixed in the spot welders. The temperature is maintained at 450–850 °C. If the time is more, it may lead to weld–decay due to formation of chromium carbides at the junction and so destroys the properties of the metals.

◎ What are the types of welds?

Cold welding is done by hammering under heavy forces so as to join the metal sheets in a coherent mass, e.g. condensation of gold foils.

Hot weld is done with the help of heat passed through the materials.

Spot weld is done under pressure on a spot welder, the electrodes of which are made of some suitable material so as to produce intense local heat and also allow the rapid dissipation of heat.

◎ What is the Elgiloy?

These are wrought Co–Cr–Ni alloy.

1. It contains 40, 20 , 15 % respectively of Co–Cr–Ni in it. And Fe is 15.8 %.
2. Age hardening is done at = 260- 650 °C range, i.e. 482 °C for 5 -hr.
3. Softening by heat Rx and quenching at = 1100–1200 °C
4. Should never be annealed.
5. Ductility = softened is > SS; hardened < SS.
6. Properties are nearly equal to = SS
7. It is of 4 types, i.e. blue / yellow / green / red elgiloys.

◎ What do you mean by Recovery heat treatment?

Stress relief heat R_x is done at 370–480 °C for 11 min, after cold working removes residual stresses.

In SS = increased MOE; increased YS; decreased ductility; increased modulus of resilience.

◎ What is the composition of Ni–Ti wires?

Ni–Ti wires = contain Ni = 54; Ti = 44; Co = 2 %. It is present in **1:1 stoichiometric ratio.**

◎ What are the important properties of this wire?

1. Shape memory / superelasticity are 2 most important properties of this wire.
2. It gives very light and continuous forces for tooth movement.
3. Austenite on heat changes to M phase; **shape memory/ superelasticity** come into play.
4. Cobalt = controls the lower transition temperature; which can be near mouth temp / 37 °C.
5. Austenite changes to M–phase under stress produces superelasticity. Additional strain is due to volume change, which results from the change in crystal structure.
6. It can not be soldered / welded.

◎ How does beta–titanium wire differ from the Ni–Ti wires?

Welding can be done in beta titanium wires.

Self Assessment Questions

1. What is the use of arch wires in orthodontics?
2. What is the composition of stainless steel alloy?
3. What do you mean by AISI series?
4. What does AISI 304 signify?
5. What is the difference between soldering and welding?

Reader's Notes

21

Tarnish and Corrosion

◎ What do you mean by tarnish and corrosion?

Tarnish = it is the surface discoloration on a metal or a loss of surface luster without any chemical change. The thin films of oxides or sulfides or chlorides are formed.

It occurs due to the formation of hard and soft deposits on the surface of restorations or by the pigment producing bacteria.

Corrosion = it's the actual deterioration of metal by reacting with the environment. It leads to disintegration of metal due to formation of various sulfides, eg hydrogen sulfide, ammonium sulfides, etc.

◎ What are the types of corrosion?

It is of 2 types:

1. Chemical / dry corrosion = here, the metal reacts to form oxides, sulfides in the absence of electrolytes, e.g. oxidation of alloy particles in the dental amalgam.
2. Electrolytic / wet corrosion = it requires the p.o. of water or other fluid electrolytes. An electrolytic cell is formed. In it, the formation of free electrons occurs. At anode, the positive ions are formed, and here occurs the corrosion due to loss of electrons or due to oxidation. But at cathode, reduction occurs and the consumption of electrons occurs here.

◎ What are the other types of corrosions?

1. Galvanic corrosion or Electro-Galvanism = it occurs in the oral cavity when 2 dissimilar metals are in direct physical contacts

with each other, e.g. Au is in contact with Ag–amalgam. Here, amalgam becomes the anode and gets corroded. An electric couple causes sharp pain ka Galvanic Shock.

2. Stress corrosion = when a metal is stressed by the cold working it becomes more reactive at the sites of maximum stresses. This becomes the anode and the corrosion starts here, e.g. in orthodontic wires.
3. Crevice corrosion or concentration–cell corrosion = electrolytic concentration cell, i.e. when a metallic restoration is partly covered by food particle the composition of electrolyte under debris will differ from the of saliva and it leads to corrosion. Oxygen concentration cell is formed due to difference in O_2 tension in b/w the parts of same filling which leads to corrosion of the restoration. More corrosion occurs where O_2 conc. is less. It occurs in narrow spaces and during micro peakage.
4. Pitting corrosion = It is the highly localized corrosion occurring on base metals such as iron, nickel and chromium, which are protected by naturally forming thin oxide films. In the presence of chlorides, this film breaks down locally and rapid dissolution of underlying metal occurs in the term of pits.

Protection against corrosion

➔ On chromium, a surface oxide film is formed and make it passive, e.g. in stainless steel.

➔ Titanium also forms a thin oxide film.

Reader's Notes

22

Functional and Orthopedic Appliances

◎ Define a myofunctional appliance?

It is defined as an appliance which causes activation of ms attached to mandible when placed in the oral cavity. And obtains its effects on the dentofacial tissues by the forces from these ms. It is also called Functional Jaw Orthopedics (FJO).

◎ What is the best age for the treatment with a functional appliance (FA) ?

- Best age for treatment with FA extends from 10 years to pubertal growth phase.
- M =12-14 years ± 1 year
- F =10-12 years ± 1 year,
- 2-3 years earlier in girls than boys.

◎ What are the main indications for use of the myofunctional appliances?

- The patient should be in the actively growing status.
- Best in horizontal growth pattern cases with a normal sized but retrognathic mandible.
- VTO should be +ve, i.e. an improvement of the facial profile should be evaluated before giving the appliance.

◎ What do you mean by the diphasic treatment?

It is the combination of the early treatment, i.e. during the active growth period; and the late treatment. The skeletal problem is treated during the active growth phase. Then after some time, the treatment of dental malpositions is done after the eruption of permanent teeth.

◎ What is the symptomatic treatment?

It is the treatment of the symptoms with which the patient reports in the dental clinic.

◎ What is the mechanism of action of the functional appliance?

With the help of a functional appliance, the mandible is placed in a forward position. This activates the muscles attached to the mandible. These ms try to come back to their original position and so apply a backward pull on the appliance. But being engaged in the upper section of the appliance, the mandible is not able to return to its original state. A downward and forward force comes into play acting on mandible.

But in turn, that force is transferred to the maxillary arch in an backward and upward direction, producing redirection of maxillary growth and the retraction of maxillary incisors; it may also cause the distalization of the maxillary molars.

◎ Explain the satisfaction of the theory of functional matrix concept with the help of myofunctional appliance therapy?

When the mandible is placed forward with the help of the functional appliances, there is an increase in space of oral cavity. Also, the tongue is placed more forward and downward. Thus the functional matrix related with this stretch of the ms of tongue and the mandible gets activated and adaptation of the bony tissues takes place according to this new position of the soft tissues.

◎ What do you mean by pterygoid response with the functional appliances?

Pterygoid response = Lateral pterygoid m. (inferior head) is affected. Checked at 6-8 weeks after start of FA therapy. When the mandible is manipulated forcefully backward, a pain is felt in this muscle, which signifies the +ve response and a successful treatment. This muscle gets adapted to a new position and its length is shortened with FA R_x.

◎ **What is meant by the head gear effect of the functional appliance?**

Head gear effect = An upward and backward force on maxilla is applied, as the mandible tries to go back to its original position under the influence of the stretched musculature. This force also prevents the maxilla from growing downward and forward. It leads to retraction of proclined incisors and distalisation/distal tipping of molars.

◎ **What is the class II elastic effect with functional appliances?**

When the mandible is placed forward and downward with the help of a functional appliance, the mandible tries to go back to its original position, as the ms attached to it get activated. That reciprocal force gets transmitted to the mandibular teeth in a forward direction and to the maxillary incisors in a backward and upward direction. This force causes the flaring of lower incisors and also helps the lingual tipping of upper incisors. This is called as the class II elastic effect.

◎ **What is the approx. amount of the force generated with a myofunctional appliance?**

Approx anterio-posterior force is 315–395 gm; and the approx vertical force is 70–175 gm depending on the vertical and the horizontal displacement of the mandible.

◎ **What should be the vertical opening with a myofunctional appliance?**

- It depends upon the amount of free way space and on the anterior facial height of the patient.
- With construction bite, bite is opened 2-3 mm beyond free way space.
- It helps to activate the ms of mandible for proper effects.

◎ **How do you determine the amount of forward placement of mandible for the correction of class II m.o.?**

It depends on the overjet values of the case. "**The rule of ten**" is followed. According to it, the total amount of vertical opening and horizontal displacement should be 10 mm. So, if vertical opening is more, the horizontal displacement should be less and vice-versa.

◎ For the correction of overjet with the help of a functional appliance, which is better, i.e. single–step advancement or partial–displacement followed by a second appliance with remaining correction?

If overjet is < 10 mm, single–step correction is indicated, with the vertical opening 2–3 mm beyond the freeway space to activate the ms.

If overjet is >10 mm, a 2-step advancement is indicated, since single advancement may jeopardize the health of the soft tissues and may be uncomfortable. According to some studies, it is better to proceed in 2-steps as it helps to activate the ms once again during the treatment.

◎ How do we achieve correction of class II molar relation with activator?

The upper teeth are allowed to erupt in the downward and backward direction, while the lower teeth erupt in upward and forward direction to allow the correction of the class II molar relation.

◎ Why the overcorrection is justified with the functional appliance therapy?

Always overcorrection is done to allow for some relapse after completion of the treatment phase, so that the required amount of correction may be achieved.

◎ Why activator is called so?

Because it activates the ms attached to the mandible. It is also called monobloc and Andresen's appliance or Norwegian appliance.

◎ What is a bionator?

It is a modification of activator in which the palatal acrylic has been replaced with coffin's spring. It also incorporates the buccinator loops to keep the cheeks away from the buccal side of the posterior teeth to help the expansion.

◎ What is the philosophy of bionator?

Bionator is based on philosophy of tongue.

◎ What is the mechanism of action of bionator?

With bionator, the mandible is displaced downward and forward in cases of Class II therapy. The coffin spring activates or stimulates the tongue in downward and forward direction, thus increasing the oral space. The buccinator loops release the pressure of buccinator ms falling on the posterior teeth and lead to expansion of the arches.

◎ What is the main function of the Coffin spring used in the bionator?

Main function of Coffin spring in bionator is to stimulate the tongue and to bring in effect FM theory concept of growth.

◎ What is the area of the operation of Frankel appliance?

FR appliance functions in vestibule of oral cavity, stretches the periosteum and causes bone growth and adaptation.

◎ What is the twin block appliance and why it is called so?

It is a myofunctional appliance. It is a 2–piece appliance separately for upper and lower arches, that is why it is called twin block appliance.

◎ What is the advantage of twin block on other functional appliances?

Twin block is better because it is a two piece appliance, is comfortable, allows complete mandibular movements without any discomfort, proper speech is possible and can be worn for 24 hr. for faster and better effects.

On what philosophy, twin block appliance is based?

It is based on the inclined plane relationship of the upper and lower posterior teeth.

◎ At what age, the appliance therapy for controlling the oral habits should be advised?

Appliance therapy to control oral habits is not recommended for children < 8 years age.

◎ What are the few examples of fixed functional appliances?

Jasper–jumper, Herbst appliance, MARS appliance, etc.

◎ What is a headgear and which are the different types of head gear?

It is an extraoral appliance, which obtains its anchorage from head region. It can be cervical / occipital / intermediate vertical type of the headgear; it is also ka low pull / medium pull / high pull head gear.

The angle of the pull is + 15 degrees to the OP for medium pull; + 45 degrees to OP for high pull and–45 degrees to OP for low pull headgear.

It can be used for orthodontic and orthopedic effects depending on the amount of the force and time of wear. For orthopedic effects, it should be used for at least 12–14 -hr/day and force used is 350–450 gm/side. It can also be used to increase the anchorage during the treatment.

◎ What is a Delaire's face mask?

- It is an orthopedic appliance used for the treatment of maxillary retrognathia, e.g. CLP, especially during the growth phase. It has a chin cup and forehead support for anchorage.
- Its modified forms are Petit's face mask; Hickham's appliance.

◎ What is the recommended age for the use of Delaire's face mask?

Best age for use of this appliance is 8–9 yrs, as the growth spurt is in action at that time and maxillary growth is in full swing. It pulls maxilla downward and forward.

◎ What is the placement of the elastics with this appliance?

- The elastics are attached from a maxillary appliance from the premolar / primary first molar region to the hooks placed at the level of oral commissure, at least 5–6 mm away from the skin.
- The force is directed downward and forward (at 15–20 degrees to OP), i.e. parallel to the normal direction of maxillary growth.

◎ RME is a recommended procedure just before the use of delaire's appliance, why?

- A phase of RME before this appliance is favorable as RME helps to activate the circum-maxillary sutures.
- It is also used in CLP patients. Its chin cup helps to control mandibular growth.
- It also helps in the forward and downward movement of the maxilla, because when RME is done, a force is generated in the backward direction. But this force is reciprocated by the pterygoid plates and the buttress, which in turn applies a forward force to the maxilla, causing its protrusion.

◎ What is a Chin cup appliance?

- It is an appliance used to control the mandibular prognathic growth. It is used in skeletal class III cases.
- It uses high pull head gear, passing just in front of the condyle.

◎ What is the main disadvantage of chin cup appliance?

- It causes lingual tipping of lower incisors under its force, which is its disadvantage.
- It may also cause traumatic changes in the condyle under heavy forces.

◎ Why a long–term retention period is required for the treatment of a prognathic mandible?

It has to be used after the treatment is over, i.e. during retention phase till the growth of mandible is over. Otherwise, the abnormal growth of mandible can again resurface and lead to relapse of the condition. It is also called Dynamic Retention.

◎ It is said that the corrective jaw surgical procedures / orthognathic surgeries should be done after the completion of the growth phase, why?

If we undertake the surgical procedures during the active growth phase, the condition may recur at a later stage since the growth is taking place according to the same abnormal pattern. The best age for orthognathic surgeries is after the completion of the active growth, i.e. after approx 18 yrs age.

Self Assessment Questions

1. How much time is normally required for R_X with FA?
2. What dento-skeletal changes can be expected with FA?
3. What is the effect of AGE during F AR_X?
4. Which FA is better – the activator or the twin block?
5. What is a twin block appliance and why it is called so?
6. What is a construction bite?
7. What are different types of C. bites?
8. What is "Rule of Ten" in C. bite formation?
9. What is clasp-knife reflex?
10. What is Biphasic R_X?
11. What is free way space and what is its average value?
12. How do you calculate FW space?
13. How do we achieve expansion with bionator?
14. How much force is required for chin-cup appliance R_X?
15. What is vertical pull HG and its effect?
16. Why activator is also called Monobloc?
17. Which are different types of FR?
18. What is the area of operation of FR?
19. What is the mechanism of action of FR?
20. What is the role of lip pads and buccal pads in FR appliances?
21. What is the philosophy behind bionator appliance?
22. What is the difference between activator and bionator appliances?

Reader's Notes

23

Cleft

◎ **What are the various Epidemiological features related to cleft of lip and palate in the human beings?**

- The incidence in India is approx. 1:800 patients, incidence increases with mother's age.
- CLP more in males than females. (M >F)
- CL is 3 times more on left side than on right. (L>R)
- Isolated CP is more common in females.
- Unilateral is more common than the bilateral CLP. (U>B)
- CL is more common in males; CP in females.

◎ **How do you classify the CLP conditions?**

- Class I = soft palate with possible notching of hard palate.
- Class II = soft and hard palate but no alveolar ridge.
- Class III = complete unilateral lip–jaw–palate cleft.
- Class IV = complete bilateral lip–jaw–palate cleft.

◎ **What is the location of cleft of alveolus and / or the CLP?**

Appears between lateral incisor and canines, generally L.I are missing.

◎ **How does the clefts of lip and /or the palate develop?**

- CL = MNP–LNP not fused = during 6th wk. i.u.
- CP = Palatal shelves not fused = during 8th wk. i.u.
- Lateral nasal process = does not contribute to (U) lip.
- Philtrum = line of fusion of MNP and maxillary process.

◎ Which embryological processes are involved in the formation of palate, upper lip and the maxilla?

- Palate is formed by maxillary process and frontonasal process (which forms premaxillary part)—(First pharyngeal arch).
- Upper lip and maxilla are formed by fusion of maxillary process with the medial and lateral nasal processes.

◎ What is "Millard's rule of 10" considered during Lip repair?

It is 10 wks age so as to assist suckling
10 lbs wt.
10 gm% Hb
10000 WBC count

◎ Why lip repair is essential at an early age?

It helps in suckling the milk and so proper diet helps to maintain the health of the child.

◎ Why palate repair is to be done at the age of 12–24 months?

It is the time of start of development of the speaking skill, i.e. child starts learning how to speak at around this age. A broken palate leads to failure in proper articulation of the words and a proper vacuum is not created for escape of air during speech.

◎ What are the disadvantages of an early repair of palate?

It leads to constriction of maxilla and improper growth of maxilla due to the scar formed by the surgery of palatal tissues.

◎ What is the recent concept of palatal repair?

It is proved that the surgery can be postponed till the completion of maxillary growth and the palatal defect can be filled by some obturator like device for proper sound development and to prevent nasal regurgitation of the food and liquids.

◎ What are different phases of orthodontics for a patient of cleft lip and palate?

A CLP patient is treated by a team of doctors. Different phases of orthodontic treatment such a patient are as follows:

- Primary dentition phase = as such no treatment is required during this stage except a cross bite condition. Parents are advised for proper feeding and hygiene of the patient.
- Mixed dentition phase = is the most important phase. Skeletal condition is treated by chin cup / face mask / expansion / myofunctional appliances etc. The teeth are guided to erupt in proper alignment. The rotations are corrected.
- Speech therapy should be given during full treatment as advised by the speech therapist.
- Primary alveolar grafting = it is to be done before the eruption of maxillary canines. A proper bony medium is required for dental eruption. So homograft is placed in the defect at around 10–11 yrs of age.
- Permanent dentition phase = the refining of the occlusion, retention of the treatment results, placement of FPD in place of missing teeth and esthetic restorations are done.
- Surgical phase = if any skeletal jaw discrepancy remains, it is removed after completion of growth by surgical methods.
- Scar refining surgeries, nasal surgery for esthetics, etc are performed.

◎ Which is the proper age of primary alveolar grafting and why?

The proper age is during the eruption of permanent maxillary canines, i.e. approx. 10–11 yrs. It is because a sound bony medium is required for the eruption of any tooth. The canine erupts at around this age.

◎ Which is the most common missing tooth in cases of cleft lip and / or palate?

It is mostly the maxillary lateral incisor, because the cleft generally passes in b/w lateral incisor and the canine, and since canine develops at a late age.

◎ What do you mean by multi-disciplinary approach and by interdisciplinary approach, and which is better?

Multidisciplinary approach means that the doctors of different specialities make a team to treat the patient. However, there is least amount of interaction b/w them.

Interdisciplinary approach means that the doctors of different specialities make a team and interact with each other and discuss the treatment plan at each step to provide the best possible treatment to the patient. It is a better approach than the former.

Self Assessment Questions

1. What is Veau's classification of clefts?
2. What do you mean by Riding Pontics?
3. Why long-term retention is required after expansion in CLP patients?
4. What is the reason behind that all possible efforts should be done to save the incisors in bilateral CLP cases?
5. Which is the appliance fabricated to block the defect of CLP in un-operated cases?
6. Which of the problems develop in untreated CLP cases?
7. What are different speech defects in CLP cases?
8. Why middle ear infections are common in CLP cases?

Reader's Notes

24

Surgical Procedures

◎ **What are different types of Surgical Procedures used in the orthodontics?**

Frenectomy, pericision, extractions, osteotomy and ostectomy, etc.

◎ **What do you mean by frenectomy?**

Frenectomy means the incising the low attached labial frenum in the upper arch, which causes midline diastema. It is also called as clipping of frenum.

◎ **Should the frenectomy be done before the diastema closure or after the closure?**

Frenum should be clipped only after orthodontic diastema closure. If it is done earlier to diastema closure, then scar elastic tissue formed there leads to relapse due to its pressure and does not allow the proper closure of the space.

◎ **What is the normal position of the upper labial frenum?**

During the gum pads stage, the frenum is normally attached in the palate near the incisive papilla. It retracts upwards with the eruption of teeth and the alveolar growth. However, in some cases, it does not retract properly and remains attached on the alveolar ridge or palate to a variable degree.

◎ **What is blanch test?**

This abnormal attachment of frenum can be tested by the blanch test. When the lip is stretched upward and outward, if the blanching occurs around the incisive papilla region, it is positive for the abnormal attachment of frenum.

◎ What is the best age for diastema closure?

Midline diastema is a normal feature during the eruption of maxillary canines, because the erupting canines slide along the lateral surfaces of roots of lateral incisors (ugly-duckling stage). So the diastema should not be attempted to close till complete eruption of canines, i.e. till 11 yrs age approx.

◎ What is the indication of lingual frenectomy?

Short lingual frenum leading to the stripping of the periodontium from the lower incisors is the indication of this procedure. It may lead to speech problems and the eating inconvenience. However, the tongue tie or the ankyloglossia does not require any treatment in many cases.

◎ What do you mean by pericision?

Rotational correction and its retention is a difficult procedure. When a tooth is derotated, the trans-septal fibers get stretched which lead to relapse. To prevent relapse, these fibers are cut till the level of alveolar crest. This process is ka **Pericision or CSF,** i.e. circumferential supracrestal fibrotomy. It was devised by Edwards.

◎ What is the minimum retention period required to avoid rotational relapse?

The minimum retention period required to avoid the rotation relapse is 232 days, which are required for readaptation of trans-septal fibers and the Alveolar Crest group of gingival fibers.

◎ What is the mechanics for rotation correction?

For correction of rotated tooth, a couple force is required. A couple is a set of 2 equal forces acting in an opposite direction and separated by a distance. This couple rotates the tooth around its vertical axis.

◎ What do you mean by bilateral sagittal split osteotomy and its indications?

In cases of mandibular hypoplasia or hyperplasia, this is a recommended procedure. It means that the ramus is splitted vertically on both sides and the mandible is either placed forward or brought backward to correct its relation with maxilla.

◎ **What other procedures can be done for the treatment of sagittal problem of mandible?**

- TOVRO, i.e. Transoral vertical ramal osteotomy;
- Reduction genioplasty for treatment of mandibular prognathism;
- Augmentation genioplasty for mandibular retognathism, etc.

◎ **Which surgery is mostly recommended for treatment of maxillary sagittal problems?**

- Lefort I osteotomy with advancement for Maxillary retrognathism.
- Lefort I osteotomy with backward placement for maxillary prognathism.
- Also, segmental osteotomy in the region of first premolar can be done for both the above problems if indicated.

◎ **What surgical procedure for treatment of short upper facial height?**

Le-Fort I with downward placement and fixing a graft in b/w is the procedure. The graft is fixed with plates.

◎ **What is the difference in orthodontic treatment planning for a patient agreeing for orthognathic surgery?**

For such a patient, the upper and lower teeth are arranged in a proper relation to their respective jaw bases, irrespective to their interocclusal relationship, as compared to the camouflage orthodontic treatment only. Also the extraction pattern differs for both the treatment plans. This phase may make the dental relations more severe than the pretreatments condition, which later on are corrected with proper surgery. So patient should be told about this before start of the treatment.

Self Assessment Questions

1. What procedure is recommended to treat a cause of increased vertical facial height?

Reader's Notes

25

Retention and Relapse

◎ **What is retention?**

It is the maintenance of the teeth in their final corrected positions after removal of the active orthodontic appliances.

◎ **What is the reason behind doing the over-treatment of each case of condition in the active phase of treatment before starting the retention phase?**

Since there is always a tendency of the teeth to come towards their original positions after completion of orthodontic treatment, even after the recommended retention period, the over-treatment is done so that the finally the teeth settle down to the acceptable positions.

◎ **What do you mean by the term RELAPSE?**

It is the loss of any correction achieved by orthodontic treatment. The teeth try to come to their original positions after the active orthodontic treatment.

◎ **What are the main causes of relapse?**

- Persistence of the cause, e.g. oral habits.
- **PDL traction** = mainly supracrestal fibers and the transeptal fibers of gingival fibers group get stretched. So, a minimum of 232 days are required for readaptation, e.g. correction of Rotations. To avoid relapse, either circumferential supracrestal fibrotomy is done OR a prolonged retention is given. PDL fibers require 4-5 months only for reorganization.

- Due to **muscular forces and occlusal imbalances.**
- Due to **growth changes**–Prolonged retention is given until active growth is complete to avoid relapse of skeletal problems (e.g. Class II, III e.g. head gear, chin cup are used. It is known as **DYNAMIC RETENTION**

◎ **Which conditions are self-retentive?**

- Treated anterior cross bites with sufficient overbite.
- Labially blocked out and upward placed canines.

◎ **Classify retention?**

It may be classified as follows:

Group	Description
I	Cases not requiring retention eg cross bite; serial extraction; highly place canine etc
II	Standard or limited retention for 3–6 months; eg class I type 2, deep bite, class II div 2
III	Prolonged retention, i.e. for > 232 days, eg rotations
IV	Permanent retention eg midline diastema; cleft palate; expansion of lower arch and severe rotations.

◎ **Why the expansion of lower arch is not stable?**

It is due to multiple factors eg Mandible is a compact bone; with no sutures and a no. of ms attached to it. An increase in intercanine width of lower arch is never stable and it always relapses. So it should not be attempted or it requires permanent retention.

◎ **Which conditions require prolonged or indefinite retention?**

- Skeletal malocclusions;
- Expansion in CLP patients
- Surgically treated skeletal discrepancies
- Midline diastema - closure, large tongue size with tongue thrusting habit, and severe rotations require PROLONGED RETENTION.

◎ **What is the cause behind the lower anterior crowding / relapse in late years of growth?**

Relapse of lower anterior crowding after growth has ceased is mainly by **LATE MANDIBULAR GROWTH** (18-25-30 years), in which mandible rotates U/F pushing the mandibular arch against the upper anterior teeth. Also 3rd molars have been implicated for it, which has been proved a wrong contention.

◎ **What is the minimum time for which the retention is required?**

Minimum time for which retention is given for a mild malocclusion is 9–12 months.

◎ **How much time is required for the readaptation of the tissues after the orthodontic treatment?**

- 3–4 months for the readaptation of periodontal fibers.
- 6–9 months for bone and trabecular adaptation.
- 9–12 months for gingival fibers arrangement.
- So main cause of relapse is the gingival fibers.

◎ **How does the condylar cartilage differs from the other joints of the body?**

It is a fibro-cartilagineous structure, rather than hyaline as in other joints.

◎ **How many bones are present in the face at birth?**

45

◎ **What is the normal age of ossification of mid-palatal suture?**

Mid palatal suture ossifies by 12-14 years.

◎ **What is the range of a normal overbite?**

Normal overbite = 33% of crowns of L.I.

◎ **What is a key-ridge?**

Key ridge = corresponds to MB root of maxillary first molar and is lowermost point on contour of anterior wall of infratemporal fossa.

◎ **What is the basic difference in the orthodontic tooth movement of a vital tooth and a root canal treated tooth?**

OTM in pulpless teeth cp. To vital teeth is the same. It is because a viable PDL is the main requirement for the proper movement of a tooth.

◎ **What is the main difference in the facial growth during puberty in males?**

Basic difference in facial growth during puberty is greater vertical development in males.

◎ **What are the various features of long face syndrome, i.e. LFS?**

1. Increased upper dental height.
2. Steep occlusal plane angle.
3. Low mandibular position with respect to the maxilla
4. Increased eruption of posterior teeth.
5. Constricted maxillary arch.
6. Skeletal open bite.
7. Incompetent lips.

◎ **What is the position of head and mandible during Mouth breathing?**

1. Forward head positioning on the neck.
2. Low mandible; low and forward placed tongue.

Self Assessment Questions

1. What are different schools of thought for retention?
2. Which factors are considered for planning the retention?
3. What do you mean by fixed retention?
4. What is the effect of growth on retention plan?
5. Why prolonged retention is required in CLP cases?
6. How does the muscular forces affect retention?
7. Which are different retention appliances?

8. Classify retainer?
9. What do you mean by lingual retainers?
10. What do you mean by bonded retainers?
11. Which is the most commonly used retainer?

Reader's Notes

A

Appendix

Chronology

1.	Maximum growth of skull completed by	6-7 years
2.	Most cranial sutures close by size of adulthood	at Birth
3.	Maximum inter canine width in mandible is completed by	9-10 years
4.	Mid-symphyseal suture fuses at age	≅ 18 mos. ≅ 2 years age)
5.	Sphenooccipital synchondrosis closes at	18-25 years
6.	Growth of Anterior cranial base completed by	6-7 years
7.	CP occurs in	8-10 week i.u.
8.	Inter canine width in maxilla completed by	10-12 years and up to 18 years (males)
9.	Maxillary sinus is first to develop and Starts develop at	4 months i.u.
10.	Papillae of tongue are seen by	11 week i.u.
11.	Taste buds in circumvallate papillae	12 week i.u.
12.	Taste buds in fungi form papillae	14 week i.u.
13.	Metopic suture of skull fuses by	5th year
14.	Ant and post fontanelles close by	1 st yr age
15.	Cleft lip and jaw would be apparent by i.u.	6th–7th week

16.	Developmental malformations of face occur during	4-12 week i.u.
17.	Union of palatine processes is completed by	3-month i.u.
18.	Greatest period of cranial growth	0-5 years
19.	Vestibule oral is apparent by	6 week i.u.
20.	Buccopharyngeal membrane persists up to	4 week i.u..
21.	Oronasal membrane ruptures at	6 week i.u.
22.	Nasobuccal membrane ruptures at	5 week i.u.
23.	Palate formation starts at and goes up to	5 -12 week i.u.
24.	Thyroglossal duct disappears by	7 week i.u.
25.	Primary and secondary ossification centres appeared at	6th week and 9 months i.u.
26.	Pharyngeal arches developed by	4th week i.u.
27.	All PNS grow rapidly at	6-7 year of age
28.	Mid palatal suture does not close until	6-7 year of age
29.	Increase in width of maxilla is mostly completed by	10-12 year of age

1.	Time of initiation of permanent first molar is (Bud develops)	4 mo i.u.
2.	Calcification of first permanent molars starts at	Birth
3.	At what age = 12 primary + 12 permanent erupted teeth	8.5 years
4.	First evidence of calcification of IInd premolars	1½–2½ years
5.	Teeth initiated after birth	4,5,7,8
6.	Jaws of newborn child show calcification of	24 teeth
7.	Enamel of permanent incisors forms between	Birth–5 years age
8.	Enamel formation/ crown formation of all primary teeth completed	by 1-11 months

9.	Time required for primary teeth to reach occlusion after cutting into oral cavity is	2-12 months
10.	Initiation of primary tooth bud is (first bud)	6 week i.u.
11.	First evidence of calcification of primary teeth	4 months i.u. (17 week i.u.)
12.	Crowns of all permanent teeth except M3 complete by	8 years
13.	Permanent tooth takes ____ years to complete apex closure after eruption	2½–3 years-
14.	Enamel formation occurs between	4 month i.u. to 12-16 years
15.	Bud of M2 starts at	1 year age
16.	Bud of M3 starts at	4-5 year age

Development of speech patterns

Speech develops from the anterior to posterior of the oral cavity.

Speech	First sounds = bilabial	m, p, b
(A→P)	Tongue tip consonants	t, d
	Sibilants	s, z
	posterior tongue positioning	r

Up to 5th year = Neurocranial dominance

After 5 years = Orofacial dominance of growth.

At this time, the mandible emerges from beneath the cranium.

Synchondroses:

- ⇒ Sphenoethmoidal = close at 5-25 year (exactly unknown)
- ⇒ Intersphenoidal = Birth
- ⇒ Sphenooccipital = 20th year = main synchondroses and **most important**
- ⇒ Inter occipital = 3-5 years

SKULL

- Skull has 45 bones at birth.
- Adult has 22 bones; these are 14 in face and 8 in the cranium.
- In the newborn, the cranium is 8–9 times larger than the facial part.
- The face makes up one fourth of the entire skeletal height at the time of birth.
- In the adult, the face makes up half the size of the cranium and the head height is reduced to one eighth of the total body height.
- Original pattern of the skull growth is maintained, with the stationary biologic center lying in the body of the sphenoid bone.

CRANIAL BASE GROWTH	Size of face : Size of body
At Birth = 55-60% of adult size	50%
4-7 years = 94% of adult size	33%
8-13 years = 98% of adult size	12%

Development of Various bones

Pure intramembranous	Frontal, zygomatic, parietal, palatal, maxilla, vomer, nasal, lacrimal
Pure endochondral	Ethmoid, Inferior nasal concha
Mixed	Mandible, occipital, sphenoid, temporal

Direction of growth

⇒ Basal cranium = U/F

⇒ Maxilla= D/F

⇒ Mandible condyle= U/B

Cranial vault	Desmocranium	**Sutural growth**
Cranial base	**Chondrocranium**	**Synchondroses**
Lower face	**Splanchnocranium**	**Membranous**

- The neurocranium follows neural type of growth.
- Lower face nearly approximates the general or bodily growth curve.

Fontanelles: there are 6 fontanelles in the skull at the time of birth. These are:

- 1 frontal
- 1 occipital
- 2 parietal
- 2 temporal

GROWTH SPURTS

	Female	**Male**
1st peak (Childhood)	3 years	3 years
2nd peak (Juvenile)	6-7 years	7-9 years
3rd peak (Prepubertal)	11-12 years	14-15 years

Intercanine width

	Maxilla	**Mandibular**
M	18 years	9-10 years
F	12 years	9-10 years

Self-correcting anomalies

GUM PADS STAGE	PRIMARY D P	MIXED D P
Open bite	Deep bite	End-on molars
Increased overjet	FTP	Ugly-duckling stage
Tongue in between gum pads	Primary spacing	< 2 mm of lower incisors crowding
	Primate spacing	
	Small mandible	
	More upright incisors	

Cephalic Index

$$I = \frac{\text{Maximum skull width}}{\text{Maximum skull length}}$$

- Dolichocephalic ×–75.9
- Mesocephalic 76–80.9
- Brachycephalic 81–85.4
- Hyperbrachycephalic 85.5–×

Differential growth rate of cranial and facial profile components

Stage \ Years age	0–5 years	5–10	10–20
Neural growth curve/cranial growth	85 % of total growth completed	96 % of total growth completed	Remaining 4% completed
Bodily growth curve/maxillary growth	45% of total growth completed	65 % of total growth completed	Remaining 35% completed
Mandibular growth/bodily growth curve	40 % of total growth completed	65 % of total growth completed	Remaining 35% completed

Morphologic Facial Index

$$I = \frac{\text{Morphologic facial height}}{\text{Bizygomatic width}}$$

Classification

- Hyper euryprosop low facial ×–78.9
- Euryprosop skeleton 79–83.9
- Mesoprosop 84–87.9
- Leptoprosop 88–92.9
- Hyperleptoprosop 93–×

Chances of the development of crowding in permanent teeth based on the crowding in deciduous teeth:

Class	In deciduous teeth	Crowding chances in permanent teeth
I	Crowded	10 in 10
II	No spaces	7 in 10
III	≤ 3 mm spacing	5 in 10
IV	3–6 mm spacing	2 in 10
V	> 6 mm spacing	None

Nolla's stages of tooth development:

0	Absence of crypt
1	**Presence of crypt**
2	Initial calcification
3	$1/3^{rd}$ crown completed
4	$2/3^{rd}$ crown completed
5	crown almost completed
6	**Crown completed**
7	$1/3^{rd}$ root completed
8	$2/3^{rd}$ root completed
9	Root almost completed, open apex
10	**Apical end of root completed**

Butler's Field Theory

According to this concept, the tooth most distal to other teeth in its field / category is the most variable in structure, form or presence. If we divide the human dentition in 4 fields, i.e. incisors, canine, premolars and molars, the lateral incisors, 2nd premolars and the 3rd molars are the most variable than their colleagues. This rule is an exception for the lower incisors region where the central incisors are more missing than the lateral incisors. Canine is the least variable tooth.

Cervical Vertebra Maturation Index

Stages	Growth expected	Shape of the cervical vertebrae	Inferior border of cervical vertebra
Initiation	80–100 %	Wedge	Flat
Acceleration	65–85 %	Rectangular	Slight concavity C2
Transition	25–65 %	Rectangular	Slight concave C3
Deceleration	10–25%	Square	Distinct concave, C2, 3
Maturation	5–10 %	Square concavity, C3	Accentuated
Completion	0–little	Vertical Dim > horizontal	Deep concavities, C 2, 3, 4

Differences

Orthodontic forces	Orthopaedic forces
Light, 50-100 gm	Heavy > 400 gm/side
Continuous	Interrupted 12-14 hr.
Dentoalveolar effects	Skeletal effects
Within physiological limits	Beyond
Compatible to the tissues	Damaging to the tissues

Forces

Forces required for tooth movements

•	Tipping	-	50 - 75 gm
•	Bodily movement	-	100 - 150 gm
•	Intrusion	-	15 - 25 gm
•	Extrusion	-	50 - 75 gm
•	Torquing	-	50 - 75 gm
•	Uprighting	-	75 - 125 gm
•	Rotation	-	50 - 75 gm
•	Head Gears	-	350 - 450 gm on each side for a minimum of 12-14 hr / day
•	Face mask	-	1 pound (450 gm) per side, (12-14 hr),
•	Chin cup two months (for 12-14 -hr.)	-	Initially 150-300 gm / side, next force is 450 - 700 gm Per side

- **Optimal force** = 20-26 gm/cm^2 root surface area (RSA). It is the force which moves the teeth most rapidly and causes no damage to tooth and associated tissues; and with minimum patient discomfort.

- Forces in expansion - SME = 2-4 lbs
  - RME = 10-20 lbs

Minimum force to be applied to cause tooth movement = 7 gm/cm^2 Minimum time for which force is to be applied to cause tooth movement = 6 hours

Different Types of Tongue Thrust

Primary	Anterior	Endogenous
Secondary	Lateral	Habitual
	Complex	Adaptive

Tongue Postures

Type I = Tongue is flat and its tip is behind the lower incisors. It is generally seen with anterior cross bite.

Type II = Tongue is flat and retracted.

RME *vs* SME

Features	RME	SME
1 **Opening**	0.5-1 mm / day (3.5-7 mm / week) 90°BD	1 mm/week 90° / 2-3 days
2 **Force generated**	10-20 lbs	2-4 lbs
3 **Tissue damage**	More	Less
4 **Skeletal : dental expansion**	8:2	5:5
5 **After 4 months of retention**	5:5	5:5

Centers of resistance of various teeth and dental and skeletal units:

C. res of single rooted tooth	In mid root region, 2/3 rd the distance from apex of the root.
C. res of molar	Bifurcation, midroot region
C. res of maxilla	Zygomatic maxillary suture
C. rot. for bodily OTM	at infinity
C. res of mandible	Apical and in between the premolars
c. Rot for root torquing	At the incisal edge of the tooth
c. Rot for controlled tipping	At the apex of the tooth

Anchorage value of teeth depends on their root surface areas (RSA)

Teeth	1	2	3	4	5	6	7
Max	230	194	282	×	254	533	450
Mano	170	200	270	×	240	475	450

Fixed Orthodontic Appliances

Plastic brackets are made of	Polycarbonate
Nitinol wires contain	Ni, Ti in 55 : 45, i.e. 1:1 stoichiometric ratio
β- titanium (TMA) contain	Ti, Mo
Elgiloy contains	Co, Cr, Ni
18:8 S.S. contains	18 Cr, 8 Ni

Elastics are made of **Latex** rubber

Class I Elastics	Intra arch, close space and retract the teeth
Class II Elastics	Inter arch, class II molar correction, retraction of (U)- anterior
Class III Elastics	Inter arch, class III molar correction, retraction of (L) anterior

(Class II, Class III also known as **Baker's anchorage**)

Box Elastics	for treatment open bite
Cross elastics	for treatment posterior cross bite
Triangular and check patterns	For occlusal settling

Various Definitions and the Basic Concepts Regarding the Orthodontics and Quick Revision Points

- **Development** = it is the growth + differentiation + translocation
- **Growth** = according to Todd, it is an increase in size.
- **Development** = it is the progress towards maturity.
- **Differentiation** = is a change from generalized cell to a specialized kind, i.e. a change in quality.
- **Translocation** = i.e. *passive* growth. It is a change in the position of whole bone. It depends on capsular matrix and is ka displacement of the bone.
- **Primary growth** = Actual **translation** (passive growth) and remodeling of bones.
- **Transformation** = it is *active growth*. It is the apposition and resorption in a bone. It is a local change and occurs under the influence of periosteal matrix, and is aka the apposition and resorption in a bone.
- **Secondary growth** = **transformation** (periosteal) + sutural growth.
- **Maturation** = it expresses the qualitative changes which occur with age.
- Bone deposition and resorption = ka **bone remodeling.**
- **Cortical drift** = it is the combination of bone deposition and resorption resulting in a growth movement towards the depository surface.
- **Displacement** = it is the movement of whole bone as a unit. It is due to pull or push of different soft and bone tissues as they all continue to enlarge.
- **Primary or active displacement** = i.e. if bone gets displaced due to its own growth. Eg growth at maxillary tuberosity pushes maxilla anteriorly.

- **Secondary or passive displacement** = i.e. if the bone gets displaced due to growth and enlargement of an adjacent bone.
- **Enlow's expanding V–principle** = many bones / parts of the bone have V–shape pattern of the growth, which occurs towards wider ends of the V due to selective apposition and resorption.
- **Enlow's counterpart principle** = states that the growth of any given facial or cranial part relates specifically to other structural and geometric counterparts in face and cranium.
- **Neurotrophism** = is a non–impulse transmitting neural function which involves axoplasmic transport and provides for long term interaction b/w neurons and innervated tissues, which homeostatically regulates the morphological, compositional and functional integrity of these tissues.

3 primary ossification centers = one above canine fossa for maxilla proper and two for premaxilla.

Basic maxillary skeletal unit = INFRAORBITAL NEUROVASCULAR TRIAD

Comparison of maxilla with the mandible:

Structures related to the developing jaws		**Developmental elements**	
Mandible	Maxilla	Mandible	Maxilla
Inferior dental nerve	Infraorbital nerve	Neural	Neural
Meckel's cartilage	Nasal capsule	Alveolar	Alveolar
Tooth germs	Tooth germs	Ramal	Zygomatic
		Muscular	Palatal
		Cartilaginous	Cartilaginous

MANDIBLE

It ossifies by **2 ossification centers,** one each in the area of future mental foramen, (appear in 6 week I.U.) lateral to Meckel's cartilage, **Ossification stops at a point which later becomes LINGULA.**

Remnants of Meckel's cartilage are malleus, incus, spine of sphenoid, sphenomandibular ligament, etc.

Lower jaw is the first to develop in the facial skeleton.

Its growth **follows GENERAL TISSUE growth curve**, while that of vault follows neural growth curve

⇒ At birth = Size of mandible arch is sufficient to accommodate all primary teeth if erupted.

⇒ 2 halves of mandible fuse by 16-18 months age.

⇒ Main growth of mandible after birth occurs at condyle, Ramus, Alveolar bone

CONDYLE

⇒ **Condyle** is the major growth CENTRE of mandible, it has **fibrocartilage** which is a secondary cartilage, grows by proliferation of cartilage. **Condyle is the only bone in body** which shows **both interstitial and appositional growth .**

Condyle grows in U and B direction - so mandible moves in D and F direction, along the arch which runs from foramen ovale to mandibular foramen to mental foramen (**unloaded nerve concept**).

⇒ **Basal tubular part** = protects mandibular nerve **(unloaded nerve concept)** and follows a logarithmic spiral in its D/F growth.

⇒ Most constant portion of mandible is the =ARC from **F. ovale to mandibular f. to mental f.**

⇒ D/F movement of mandible is primarily *passive translation.*

⇒ **Active transformation** = minor D/F changes but mainly U/B compensatory growth. of ramus.

⇒ Condyles are not primary site of mandibular growth, but are loci with secondary, compensatory growth potential.

RAMAL GROWTH

⇒ In infancy = the ramus is located at approx. primary first molar area.

Growth occurs along the **V-principle**. Anterior border is resorptive to provide space for eruption of permanent molars. After 6 years age, greatest increase in size of mandible occurs distal to first molars. Posterior surface is depository.

Ramal growth **provides space vertically** in which both U/L alveolar bones grow, the teeth being their functional matrices.

LATE MANDIBULAR GROWTH—occurs in horizontal direction and is mainly responsible for lower anterior crowding, rather than mandibular third molars, which appears, develops or increases in the adult age/ post pubertal age (20-30 years age.)

⇒ (L) incisors tend to upright under the terminal horizontal growth increments, which occurs due to U and F rotation of mandible, leading to lingual movement of lower incisors.

ALVEOLAR GROWTH

Distance between mental foramina = changes little after 6 years age (i.e. width of mandible).

Mental foramen level changes with growth, from near mandibular border (infants) to middle of the body (in adults) to at alveolar crest (in edentulous patient)

Level of mandibular foramen lies below OP in children and at the level of OP in adults.

CRANIUM: DW (H) (i.e. growth in D is most rapid, with growth in W and H in that order)

FACE: HD (W)

H shows greatest incremental changes with age

W shows least incremental change with age

⇒ So **at birth, Height of cranium and width of face are closest to adult size.**

⇒ Growth is generally completed first in head, then in W of face and last in L (D) of face

⇒ female pubertal spurt occurs 2-3 yrs ahead of that of male.

THEORIES OF GROWTH: most important is **functional matrix theory by Moss.**

FCC

Functional matrix	Skeletal unit
• Periosteal matrix	1. Macroskeletal unit
	2. Microskeletal unit
• Capsular matrix	
1. Neurocranial capsule	
2. Orofacial capsule	

⇒ Major difference in the theories is the LOCATION at which genetic control is expressed.

⇒ Indirect genetic control is known as EPIGENETIC.

⇒ **SITE**= is a location where growth occurs

⇒ **CENTER** = is a location **at which independent, genetically controlled growth occurs,** i.e. independent of environment.

⇒ 2 capsular matrices—neurocranial and orofacial

Growth Spurts

	Females	Males
1st peak (Childhood)	3 years	3 years
2nd peak (Juvenile)	6-7 years	7-9 years
3rd peak (Prepubertal)	11-12 years	14-15 years

Inference

⇒ More boys to have 2-3 peaks

⇒ Girls show only 2 peaks

⇒ V. few girls show MDP growth spurt, but all show pubertal growth spurt.

⇒ So MDP jaw changes (with FJO) is more successful in boys.

⇒ Female mature earlier (2-3 years) than males, so early treatment is more critical in girls than in boys.

⇒ During pubertal growth period = there is directional change from Vertical to- Horizontal.

CLINICAL IMPLICATIONS

1. Intercanine width

	Maxilla	Mandibular
M	18 years	9-10 years
F	12 years	9-10 years

2. Maxillary inter canine width is a **SAFETY VALVE** - when the final horizontal growth of mandible especially in males, causes a forward movement of mandibular base with teeth.

⇒ In both M, F = Maxillary intercanine dimension serves as a *safety valve* for pubertal growth spurt, where basal horizontal mandibular growth partly unmatched by maxilla, as mandible grows D and F.

⇒ Onset of menstruation = growth spurt is all but complete.

3. growth modulation therapy is better and results are stable, if given during the spurts period.

GROWTH COMPLETION SEQUENCE

1) W = Both jaws + arches = before adolescent growth. spurt especially on canine regions, but in M2/M3 region, width increases due to jaws growth in length posteriorly.
2) D (Length) = continues through period of puberty

   F = 14-15 years (2-3 years after menstruation)

   M = approx. 18 years (4 years after sexual maturity)
3) H in Female = 17-18 years and in M = early 20's

General Facts about the growth

- Bone tissues grow by = appositional growth change
- Condyle of mandible grows by = proliferation of cartilage
- Cartilage grows by = both interstitial and appositional growth
- Bone tissues grow by = differentiation of cartilagineous tissues
- Cartilage differs from bone in that = cartilage grows by interstitial growth.
- Long bones grow in length by = interstitial growth in cartilagineous epiphyseal plate.
- In endochondral ossification = the calcified cartilage is replaced by bone. The function of hyaline cartilage is to provide a region where bone can grow in length.

Development of Dentition

Primary spacing/ physiological /developmental spacing—occurs due to growth, helps in proper alignment of bigger size permanent teeth, 70% in maxilla and 63% in mandible.

Primate/simian/anthropoid spaces are found mesial to primary maxillary canines and distal to primary mandibular canines, named as it is found in primates, i.e. between BC/ CD.

A. MIXED DENTITION PERIOD

Begins with the eruption of first permanent molars at 6 yeas of age., generally in end-on relationship marks the Stage I of natural bite opening.

First transitional period/ early MDP—eruption of 6,1,2, mostly lower erupt first, 6-8 years age.

Correction of FTP/end on relation to class I occurs by utilization of physiologic space, leeway space and differential forward growth of the mandible.

Early mesial shift occurs in **open dentition at 6-7 years** , due to closure of primate spaces by pressure of erupting molars.

Late mesial shift occurs **in closed dentition at 10-11 years** , due to closure of leeway spaces after shedding of primary second molars.

Incisal liability—difference between sizes of primary and permanent incisors, 7 mm in upper and 5 mm in lower arch, overcome by–utilization of interdental spacing, incisor inclination labially, increased intercanine width. **(Warren Mayne's principles) as given in the table.**

Method	Maxilla	Mandible
I/D spacing	0 –10 mm, av. = 4 mm	0–6 mm, av. = 3 mm
Increase in intercanine width	4.5 mm	3 mm
Incisor position	2.2 mm	1.3 mm

⇒ **Incisor liability**: Difference in size of permanent and primary teeth, space comes from 3 sources:

1. *Increase intercanine width* = 2 mm, M>F, U>L
   Girls have greater liability to incisor crowding
2. *Labial positioning* of permanent incisors = 1-2 mm
3. *Repositioning* of mandibular canines distally in primate spaces when mandibular Lower Incisors erupt = 1 mm space. (But not in (U) arch, as primate space is between B and C.

⇒ In primary dentition - An equivalent of Class III is never seen, due to growth pattern of mandible, which lags behind the maxilla.

⇒ **Also C2 D2 is not seen in primary dentition.**

⇒ If a child has FTP in MDP, then approx. 3.5 mm of movement of mandibular first molar forward with respect to maxillary first molar is required for smooth, transition to class I relation in permanent DP, i.e. a one half cusp transition in molar relation.

Inter-transitional period–is a quite period, 8—10 years of age, no change in dentition occurs.

Late mixed dentition / second transitional period — eruption of 3,4,5,: leeway space of Nance is the difference between MD sizes of CDE and 345; 1.8 mm in maxilla and 3.4 mm in mandible.; mostly due to primary mandibular second molar ka E–space (2–3 mm), helps in late mesial shift to achieve class I molars.

Space age = is MDP

Pronounced attrition in MDP is observed to help in decrease in deep bite, prevent interlocking and thus paving way to unhindered forward growth of mandible.

Deep bite decreases by eruption of permanent molars, attrition of incisors and forward movement of mandible due to growth.

Intercanine width increases more in spaced dentition, more in maxilla, up to a later age in maxilla.

Secondary spacing occurs in closed dentition, with eruption of lower incisors which pushes primary mandibular canine laterally. It creates space for proper eruption of maxillary lateral incisors. It helps to increase the intercanine width in both arches and increase in arch circumference in maxilla.

Ugly duckling stage of Broadbent: In maxillary, 8-9 years age, canines pressing roots of laterals, root crowding, crowns move distally, spaces develop, should not be disturbed till eruption of canines, is a self correcting anomaly.

Arch length decreases by 2–3 mm when MDP changes to PDP, both from anterior and posterior sides. Also posterior teeth move mesially throughout life due to attrition and anterior component of force.

Largest arch length = is before eruption of first permanent molar.

Signs of incipient malocclusion are –lack of interdental spacing in primary dentition, crowding in permanent incisors in MDP and premature loss of primary canines especially mandibular.

Transition in chewing pattern develops in conjunction with eruption of permanent canines at age 12 years.

⇒ Owen says = Space loss (due to caries) is most likely in mandibular deciduous second molar area.

⇒ **Chewing pattern of child Vs adult -** adult opens straight and then lateral / child moves laterally.

Natural bite opening –at 6,12, 18 years of age , with eruption of permanent molars.

⇒ 3 periods of bite opening (Schwarz)

⇒ 6 years =when Ist molar erupts,12 years = 2nd molar molar erupts,18 years = 3rd molar molar erupts.

⇒ U/L permanent incisors erupt lingual to primary teeth and move forward under the tongue pressure as they erupt.

⇒ 7-8 years age = critical period

⇒ sudden change during the eruption of the CI and LI is shown by = **1.5 mm Crowding** in both M and F. Average female recovers slightly better than males.

⇒ No great relief of crowding in incisor region is expected after full eruption of L.I.

⇒Maxillary CI seem to erupt from LABIAL
⇒Mandibular. CI, LI seem to erupt from LINGUAL
⇒Maxillary. L.I. = no labial gingival bulge.
⇒maxillary second molar erupts D and F
⇒maxillary third molar erupts D and B and outward

⇒ Axial inclination of Maxillary teeth tend to converge apically especially at the end of the arch and mandibular axes tend to diverge following the C.O. Spee.

CLINICAL APPLICATIONS

⇒ Most crowding = (L) anterior segments

⇒ Occlusal contact is only 2-6% in 24 -hr. period.

⇒ Primary incisors are more vertical and intrinsical angle is more greater causing deep bite.

⇒Maxillary 2 are displaced generally LINGUALLY.
⇒Maxillary 3 are displaced generally LABIALLY
⇒Maxillary 5 are displaced generally PALATALLY.

Cephalic Index : Breadth × 100/ Width

- Dolichocephalic: 75 or less
- Mesocephalic : 75-80
- Brachycephalic: 80 or more

Important points

Step child of dentition	3rd molars
Corner stone of the dentition	First molars
Corner tooth of the dentition	Canines
Servant of the tooth	Alveolar process
Bed of the OTM	PDL
Slave of the orthodontist	Alveolar bone
Bread of the orthodontist	PDL
Cranial base	Chondrocranium
Cranial vault	Desmocranium
Cranial cavity	Neurocranium
Maxilla	Splanchnocranium

Forces in the different conditions

Condition	Male	Females
Open bite	97 lbs	96 lbs
Deep bite	118 lbs	104 lbs

Cast Analysis

1. Ashley Howe's analysis

If PMBAW

≤ 37%	Extraction
37-44%	Border Line
> 44%	Non-Extraction

2. Bolton's Analysis

⇒ Anterior Ratio = 77.2%

⇒ Overall Ratio = 91.3%

3. Peck and Peck Ratio

(L) C.I. = 88-92%

(L) L.I. = 90-95%

4. Proffit's space analysis

If TSALD is 0–5 mm	=	non-extraction case
5–9 mm	=	Borderline case
> 9 mm	=	Extraction case

5. Carey's analysis

If crowding is 0–2.5 mm	=	non extraction case
2.5–4 mm	=	second premolar extraction case
more than 4 mm	=	first premolar extraction case

Ideal cases for serial extraction are;

- 8½ - 9½ year age (Growing period)
  TSALD≥ 10 mm
- Skeletal Class I relations
- but it causes lingual tipping and deep bite development.

Various technical points of cephalometry

- Acceptable magnification on ceph its 5-7% (80 KV/8mA/ 0.8 sec.)

- Distance of film from midsagittal plane in ceph = 18 cm
- Distance of X-ray source to midsagittal plane = 5 Feet
- Mainly LHS of ceph in taken
- Jarabak ratio = PFH/AFH % = 62-65%
- Ratio of AUFH to ALFH is = 45 : 55 or 1 : 1.2
- Bjork's sum = NSAr + SArGo + arGoMe = 396° ± 6°
- Tweed's triangle includes FMA, FMIA and IMPA.
- Normal interincisal distance = 40-45 mm

Various soft tissue lines are = (MRSH)

- Merrifield's line = line passing from soft tissue pognion to the most prominent lip, whether upper or lower.
- Rickett's line = line passing from soft tissue pognion to the tip of the nose.
- Steiner's line = line passing from soft tissue pognion to the centre of the S- shaped curve formed by passing from nose to the upper lip.
- Holdaway's line = line passing from soft tissue pognion to the most prominent point on upper lip.

Hand wrist R/G

- Absence of sesamoid bone at average onset of puberty in a female => retardation of pubertal development.
- Initiation ossification of pisiforms and hook of hamate = preceded peak growth in most males and females.
- Initial ossification of thumb and advanced ossification of HH coincided with peak growth in most M and that was true in only about half of the F.

Methods of gaining space:

- Expansion = 1 mm / mm of expansion can be gained in intercanine region.
- Reproximation = 0.5 mm per interdental area, i.e. 0.25 mm per tooth surface.

- Distalisation of molars = up to 5-6 mm space can gained on each side of the upper arch. It is not possible in lower arch, where only distal tipping is achieved.
- Protrusion of incisors = 1 mm / mm of protrusion can be gained, i.e. 0.5 mm / side of the arch.
- Derotation of molars / PMs = rotated posteriors occupy more space.
- Uprighting of incisors = MD inclined anteriors occupy more space.
- Uprighting of molars
- Extraction = 7 mm / side of space can be gained by removal of first premolars.

Stripping indicated if TSALD = 0-2.5 mm

- Not > 50% enamel thickness should be reduced, i.e. 0.25 mm / surface
- Immediate Fluoride application is recommended to replenish the surface layer of enamel with Fluoride.
- ARS, i.e. air rotor stripping is better than the hand strips.

FORCES

Type of forces

1. **Continuous**
   - e.g. light wire appliance
   - Very light force
   - Direct resorption
   - No rest period
   - Decrease little in magnitude
2. **Intermittent,** e.g. removable appliance
   - Become zero with time
   - High forces
3. **Interrupted forces,** e.g. Headgears, FA
   - Heavy forces (200-300 gm)
   - Used for 12-14 hr / day
   - Become zero abruptly when appliances are removed

⇒ Main fibers affected during OTM and most abundant are OBLIQUE FIBRES.

PHASES OF OTM

- Very rapid OTM = In Initial phase, by compressed PDL.
- Little / no OTM = In lag phase, DUE TO HYALINISATION
- Rapid OTM = In post- lag phase, due to removal of hyalinised areas

⇒ **First messengers** in OTM = PTH, PG, Subs P, VIP

⇒ **2nd messengers** in OTM= CAMP, CGMP, Ca^{2+}

⇒ **step child of dentition =** third molars

⇒ **corner stone of the dentition =** first molars

⇒ **corner tooth =** canines

⇒ **servant of the tooth =** alveolar process

⇒ **bed of OTM =** PDL

⇒ D and F pull of headgear force (15-20° to OP) is applied (450 gm/side for 12-14 -hr/day

⇒ Orthodontic force should be light and gentle for rapid OTM and should be 1-2 OZ.

⇒ Light continuous forces are better and preferred and cause **frontal resorption.**

⇒ Heavy forces cause **rear resorption , undermining resorption**.

⇒ PGE1 palys role in OTM (arachidonic acid metabolites)

⇒ NSAIDS, i.e. Brufen, etc. inhibit OTM as they interfere with production of prostaglandins.

CHARACTERISTICS OF WIRES: Longer / thinner wires decrease the load-deflection rate and provide a more gentle force system.

STRENGTH	=	STIFFNESS X RANGE.
D3/L	=	D4/L3 X L2/D
SPRIGINESS	=	1/ STIFFNESS

ANCHORAGE

- Simple - Resistance to tipping
- Stationary - Resistance to bodily OTM
- Reciprocal - Tooth move equal and opposite
- Minimum - > 1/2 space can be lost by mesial movement of the anchor teeth.
- Moderate - 1/4 to 1/2 space can be lost by mesial movement of the anchor teeth.
- Maximum - < 1/4 space can be lost by mesial movement of the anchor teeth.
- Hammock - By PDL
- Muscular - By lower lip, e.g. lip bumper, etc.
- Cortical - By mandibular cortex (Rickett's)
- Extraoral Anchorage = HG
- Intra oral Anchorage = Elastics, TPA, LHA, NPA, More number of teeth involved
- Baker's Anchorage = Class II, III elastics
- Single /primary anchorage = only one tooth acts as anchorage
- Compound anchorage = more than one tooth acts as anchorage
- Reinforced / multiple anchorage = where more than one type of resistance unit is used.
- Anchorage loss is more in maxilla than mandible, due to more cancellous bone in maxilla.
- Mandibular teeth provide better anchorage than maxillary teeth due to dense bone and direction of trabeculae.
- Anchorage savers = HG, TPA, LHA, NPA, etc.

EXPANSION

Pitch of screw = 360°, i.e 0.8 mm

Expansion schedule: SME = 90° / 3 days

RME = 90° / BD

Fixed Expansion by Coffin, Haas, Hyrex, quad helix, w-arch, bihelix, NPE.

EXTRACTIONS in orthodontics

⇒ **Wilkinson's extraction** = Removal of all first permanent molars, at 8½ - 9 ½ years age

⇒ **Stobie's extraction** = removal of ADJACENT premolars at one time.

⇒ **Therapeutic extraction** = Removal of teeth for treatment - purpose.

⇒ **Balancing** = Removal of teeth from both sides in same arch

⇒ **Compensating** = Removal of teeth from same side in both arches.

⇒ **Serial extraction** = removal of CD4. It is also known as the GUIDANCE OF THE ERUPTION.

⇒ Serial extraction causes **deepening of bite**, due to lingual inclination and uprighting of lower incisors.

Reader's Notes

READER'S RESPONSE FORM

Readers are requested to fill the following form and mail it to us giving their invaluable suggestions about the strength and weaknesses of this book for further improvement of the future editions and volumes of this book. The successful students are also requested to contribute generously their ideas and notes for inclusion in further editions of this series for the benefit of their younger friends preparing for the PG entrance examinations. The criticism from the fellow readers and students will be highly appreciated.

1. **Name and address of the student:**
2. **Qualification:**
3. **Phone No. and E-mail i.d:**
4. **Good points about the book:**
5. ______________________________

6. **Problems faced while studying this book:**

7. **Experience of successful candidates while preparing:**

8. **Missing points / topics in this book:**

9. **Contributions from the students in the form of tables, MCQs, latest patterns of exams in different states etc:**

THANKING ALL OF YOU IN ANTICIPATION.

Please mail the completed form to:

Dr. Sandeep Goyal, Reader, Department of Orthodontics and Dentofacial Orthopedics, MM College of Dental Sciences and Research Mullana, Ambala, Haryana